000933

D1144940

# SOCIAL STRESS IN DOMESTIC ANIMALS

# Current Topics in Veterinary Medicine and Animal Science

Volume 53

For a list of titles in this series see final page of this volume.

# Social Stress in Domestic Animals

A Seminar in the Community Programme for
the Coordination of Agricultural Research,
held in Brussels, Belgium, 26-27 May 1988

Sponsored by the Commission of the European
Communities, Directorate-General for Agriculture,
Coordination of Agricultural Research

Edited by

## R. ZAYAN

Department of Experimental Psychology
and IRSIA, Université Catholique de Louvain,
Louvain-la-Neuve, Belgium

and

## R. DANTZER

Psychobiology Unit,
INSERM-INRA,
University of Bordeaux II,
Bordeaux, France

KLUWER ACADEMIC PUBLISHERS

DORDRECHT/BOSTON/LONDON

FOR THE COMMISSION OF THE EUROPEAN COMMUNITIES

ISBN 0–7923–0615–5

---

Publication arrangements by
Commission of the European Communities
Directorate-General Telecommunications, Information Industries and Innovation,
Scientific and Technical Communications Unit, Luxembourg

EUR 11710
© 1990 ECSC, EEC, EAEC, Brussels and Luxembourg

Published by Kluwer Academic Publishers,
P.O. Box 17, 3300 AA Dordrecht, The Netherlands.

Kluwer Academic Publishers incorporates the publishing programmes of
D. Reidel, Martinus Nijhoff, Dr W. Junk and MTP Press.

Sold and distributed in the U.S.A. and Canada
by Kluwer Academic Publishers,
101 Philip Drive, Norwell, MA 02061, U.S.A.

In all other countries, sold and distributed
by Kluwer Academic Publishers Group,
P.O. Box 322, 3300 AH Dordrecht, The Netherlands.


*Printed on acid-free paper*

Printed in the Netherlands

CONTENTS

PREFACE

Social stress in domestic animals, with particular reference to farm livestock, was the topic of a workshop held on May 26-27, 1988 in Brussels, at the Commission of the European Communities, Directorate General for Agriculture. Obviously, the problem of stress bears direct relevance to the issue of physiological and mental suffering of animals raised in large groups for industrial production. The purpose of the meeting was not to contribute to a better understanding of animal stress in general. This objective was superbly achieved by another Community workshop, the proceedings of which were recently published in another volume of the same collection. This volume, edited by Wiepkema and Van Adrichem (1987), provides an integrative approach to stress, viewed as a complex biological state tackled from several fields of research: endocrinology, immunology, pathology, neurobiology, and modelling some of the internal states involved in stress. Admittedly, the central question in most discussions was the meaning of the concept of stress; as a general rule, it was meant to refer to "the individual response state evoked by stressors". It was also emphasized that there are psychological stressors in addition to physical ones, an assertion that apparently led to discuss many of the "cognitive and emotional processes in the organisms involved".

Interestingly, some of the contributions to be found in the present volume are specifically devoted to these psychobiological components of stress. Various aspects of social recognition were systematically investigated,

vii

because the classical literature on social stress contains the inescapable statement that social tension is reduced among familiar conspecifcs, whereas the grouping of strangers will cause conflict and aggression. However, what makes the specificity of the present contributions in their attempt to circumscribe precise contexts in which _social_ stress occurs. Particular reference to social behaviour and to social structure was already made in a previous volume devoted to the spatial requirements of domestic animals, and edited by one of us in the same collection (R. Zayan, 1985). Incidentally, another factor classically acknowledged as a cause of social stress, namely crowding, typically concerns the area of social space. But a more fundamental reason similarly motivated the organization of the two workshops. Much of the applied research on social space consisted of a great deal of correlations showing that as density increased, aggression tended to increase, whereas production and health tended to decrease. However, very little experimental work had been carried out in order to control for the respective effects of group size and of available floor area per individual, since these two density variables were most often confounded in the earlier literature. In the case of social stress, too, negative influences of crowding and of aggression among strange conspecifics have been repeatedly and consistently assessed upon production, growth or health. But the specificity of the causal factors (i.e. the supposed social stressors), the precise nature and diversity of the stress responses, and the possible mechanisms leading from stressful inputs to modifications in the behavioural and physiological outputs, still remain to be delineated. Some progress would already be achieved if the complexity of social stress was to appear more clearly to all those wishing to conduct research in this field. As will hopefully also appear, such complexity requires an integrative, or multilevel. approach trying to understand how a group's social structure may induce physiological stress in individuals, via their behavioural interactions and the psychological processes that mediate the latter. Needless to say, reductionism has no future in a field as complex as social stress. Such complexity has so much inspired one of the editors that he must apologize for having written the two longest papers of the volume. He hopes to be forgiven by the contributors responsible for the shorter papers, because one needs much space to review the many problems raised by past as well as by future research on social stress. Time and space were also needed to interpret a great deal of experimental research involving behavioural observations, hormonal measures and cognitive hypotheses about the control of social stress in pigs.

R. Zayan and R. Dantzer.

REFERENCES

Wiepkema, P.R. and Van Adrichem, P.W.M. (Editors) 1987. Biology of Stress in Farm Animals: An integrative Approach. Martinus Nijhoff Publishers for the C.E.C.

Zayan, R. (Editor) 1985. Social Space for Domestic Animals. Martinus Nijhoff Publishers for the C.E.C.

GENERAL INTRODUCTION

SOCIAL STRESS: A NEW FIELD OF RESEARCH IN DOMESTIC ANIMALS

The concept of social stress has a peculiar semantic status. On the one hand, it is often understood as a patchwork notion: it encompasses all the confusions raised by the concept of physiological stress, but also the fuzziness many constipated physiologists attribute to anything that belongs to the galaxy, inaccessible to them, of "social behaviour". On the other hand, social stress is vaguely understood as any cause of stress associated with the presence of conspecifics in the immediate environment of animals. A typical example of such unspecific social stressor is crowding. Another is the mixing of unfamiliar conspecifics, known to elicit aggression. In classical experiments with domestic fowl, social "tension" was induced in the members of stable peck-orders by placing a strange intruder in their home pen. In a nutshell: social stress would coincide with aggression, and agonistic experience would induce physiological responses typical of stress.

This volume attempts to go beyond these traditional views. In a certain way, it complements and expands many of the contributions published in another book of the same collection (Zayan, 1985), in which many aspects of crowding were dealt together with density variables, i.e. increase in group size and/or reduction in floor area available per individual.

In the same volume, Dantzer and Raab (1985) have discussed the many difficulties raised by the interpretation of the behavioural and physiological correlates of social density, ranging from social isolation to crowding. The authors have rightly questioned the common belief that crowding

xi

induces stress preferentially in the subordinate members of a population of domestic animals. They also have critically examined some of the literature on physiological stress in animals of different social status, pointing to some equivocal findings. For example, whereas in pairs of male mice subordinates show higher plasma corticosterone titers than dominants, the plasma corticosterone levels of male Japanese quails do not differ in the winners and in the losers of short-term dyadic encounters. In cattle, corticosteroid levels may not be correlated with social rank, or may not be significantly modified by experimental changes in social rank; in pigs, more pronounced plasma cortisol levels are found in losers than in winners of paired encounters among unfamiliar individuals. Results such as these suggest that plasma corticosteroid levels might actually be increased by fighting, a stressful experience, but would not consistently reflect the stressful experience of losing a fight. As a matter of fact, aggression is often confused with the outcomes of aggressive encounters, i.e. dominance or subordination. Such confusion does not seem to considerably undermine the conclusions about changes in plasma testosterone levels, which appear as a reliable indicator of aggressiveness, and as such tend to increase both in aggressive and in dominant individuals. But corticosteroid levels may not provide a reliable indicator of aggressive stress, let alone of social stress in general, even if positive correlations were found between the amount of aggressive behaviour and plasma corticosterone levels in rats fighting in pairs. Firstly, the winners of fights might be just as stressed in maintaining their status as are the losers in being constantly constrained by their dominants. Secondly, there is no straightforward relation between the amount of aggression manifested during fights and the probability of winning or losing fights. Eventual subordinates often manifest more agonistic activities (i.e. both aggression and flight responses), so that they may more often experience social fear during encounters, And, as noted by Dantzer and Raab, plasma corticosteroids were not found to be higher in male birds engaged in territorial fights than in non-aggressive individuals. In already defeated animals, plasma testosterone levels are decreased and corticosterone levels are increased, the submissive behaviours being facilitated by glucocorticoids and the aggressive behaviours being simultaneously inhibited. The fact, however, that dominants sometimes have higher pituitary - adrenal activity than subordinates, led to the suggestion that neither aggression nor the aggressive outcomes directly activate the pituitary - adrenal axis. Stress may actually result from cognitive or psychological processes by which agonistic events are perceived as a source of potential danger that forces the animal to make extreme adjustments in its physiology and/or behaviour in order to cope with it.

To summarize the situation: the field of research on social stress still needs to inquire about the precise causal factors of stress, about the nature of the behavioural and physiological responses to alleged social stressors, and about the mechanisms that ensure adaptation to social causes of acute or of chronic stress.

The same as with stress in general, social stress must somehow serve a function other than coping with adverse stimuli emanating from conspecifics. Positive aspects of stress were rightly envisaged by several authors, e.g. by Freeman (1987) who referred to Amoroso's (1967) definition of stress as "a set of Situations That Release Emergency Signals necessary for Survival". But survival requires, at least in many species forming stable groups, the

xiv

presence and actions of conspecifics, so much so that separation or
disruption of social contact is often considered as a cause of stress in
domestic animals. A social context is, therefore, both a potential cause of
stress and the main reason why individuals keep together, sometimes against
their own immediate interest. This is particularly the case with highly
gregarious species such as domestic fowl. No social system would be formed,
be it a large society of just a pair of conspecifics, without some
cooperation that keeps animals connected, even when competition temporarily
induces stress to increase the resource gain of individuals. Sometimes,
group membership even coincides with animals coping together with a common
stressful situation. So, to understand what reduces social stress is at least
as essential as to disclose specific social stressors.

Social familiarity is one of the basic factors that maintains cooperation
and increases the mutual advantage of group-members in the presence of a
danger. In contrast to competition, cooperation requires that conspecifics
be known to each other before they attempt to solve a conflict (Axelrod,
1984). Where there is mutual benefit and cooperation, we find familiar
animals communicating by small and subtle signals, and avoiding overt
fighting even when there appears to be conflict (Dawkins, 1985; Zayan, 1987).
For example, crowding may not necessarily result in aggressive tension; as
with artifical confinement, groupmates may cope with it by deciding to share
the available space (Zayan et al., 1983). In contrast, temporary separation
and social strangeness cause stress or increase sensitivity to environmental
stress.

These are, thus, at least three levels at which social structure can
induce stress: - that of sudden isolation or of prolonged separation of pair-

members or of group-members; - that of social strangeness of conspecifics meeting for the first time as pair-members; - that of social instability of the relations between conspecifics forming at least triads, for the latter are the minimum subsets of a complete social system (for example, the transitive dominance relations that characterize a linear dominance hierarchy require at least three dyadic relations). In all cases, social stability is perhaps the key concept to understand how social stress originates. And, together with social cohesion or integration, social stability is an emergent property of social systems (at least dyads); it is not possessed by any of its components (individual conspecifics), let alone by subsystems of the latter (intra-individual organic processes). So, genuine explanations of social stress require a multilevel approach. This integrative perspective is based upon certain principles such as the following.

- The emergent properties of a social system, in particular those of the social structure developed by the group members, affect the latters' behaviour and physiological responses. Thus, the relative instability e.g. of a dominance hierarchy determines the disposition of each group-member to perceive social events as stressors and to respond to these by physiological stress.
- The nature, frequency and intensity of the behavioural interactions among the pair-members forming a group correspond to other interindividual connections that are not directly observable. They constitute the set of psychological couplings, and they actually control (i.e. facilitate or inhibit) the occurrence of the behavioural interactions; these social couplings are cognitive and emotional processes. Thus, aggression may be elicited by the detection of a strange conspecific in the group, but it will

be considerably reduced by recognition among familiar individuals. Similarly, strangeness may induce social fear or aversion, and recognition may induce social attraction or preference for certain individuals.

- The behavioural interactions and the psychological couplings, observed or inferred at the interindividual level, are controlled by internal states of the connected individuals. Thus, aggression by the "stressor" animal corresponds to hormonal indicators of aggressiveness, whereas the flight responses by the "stressed" animal correspond to hormonal indicators of social fear. However, the main difference between stress, an individual state (actually a process) and social stress, an interindividual process, is that in the latter the behavioural, the psychological and the physiological events of each individual have to be related to the corresponding events in the other individual(s). Ideally, such relation should be a lawful one and be expressed as a mathematical function. An integrative approach to stress in domestic animals has already been proposed, though mainly from the viewpoint of biological control (Wiepkema and Van Adrichem, 1987). The present volume being devoted to social stress, it is hoped that it will help to develop a more sociologically oriented integrative approach to the problem of coping with conspecifics.

R. Zayan and R. Dantzer

## REFERENCES

Amoroso, E.C. 1967. Discussion. In "Environmental Control in Poultry Production" (ed. T.C. Carter). Oliver and Boyd.

Axelrod, R. 1984. The Evolution of Cooperation. Basic Books.

Dantzer, R. and Raab, A. 1985. On the interpretation and significance of behavioural and physiological indicators of stress related to social space in domestic animals. In "Social Space for Domestic Animals" (ed. R. Zayan). Martinus Nijhoff Publishers for the C.E.C., pp. 3-14.

Dawkins, M.S. 1985. Social space: the need for a new look at animal communication. In "Social Space for Domestic Animals" (ed. R. Zayan). Martinus Nijhoff Publishers for the C.E.C., pp. 15-22.

Freeman, B.M. 1987. The stress syndrome. World Poult. Sci. J., 43, 15-19.

Wiepkema, P.R. and Van Adrichem, P.W.M. (Editors) 1987. Biology of Stress in Farm Animals: An Integrative Approach. Martinus Nijhoff Publishers for the C.E.C.

Zayan, R. (Editor) 1985. Social Space for Domestic Animals. Martinus Nijhoff Publishers for the C.E.C.

Zayan, R. 1987. Spatial indicators of individual recognition in laying hens. In "Cognitive Aspects of Social Behaviour in the Domestic Fowl" (eds. R. Zayan and I.J.H. Duncan). Elsevier Scientific Publishing Co., pp. 439-492.

Zayan, R., Doyen, J. and Duncan, I.J.H. 1983. Social and space requirements for hens in battery cages. In "Farm Animal Housing and Welfare" (eds. S.H. Baxter, M.R. Baxter and J.A.D. Mac Cormack). Martinus Nijhoff Publishers for the C.E.C., pp. 67-90.

SESSION I : GENERAL BACKGROUND

# THE CONCEPT OF SOCIAL STRESS

## R. DANTZER

INRA-INSERM U.259
Psychobiologie des Comportements Adaptatifs
Rue Camille Saint-Saëns
33077 Bordeaux Cedex - France

## ABSTRACT

The concept of social stress expresses the fact that social factors have adverse influences on behaviour and physiology of subordinate or crowded animals. This concept is unable, however, to account for the diversity of social influences on physiological functions such as reproduction and, in addition, its use tends to shadow more positive aspects of life in social groups, such as the buffering effects of the presence of social companions on reaction to environmental stressors. For these various reasons, the use of the term social stress should be avoided and a more thorough evaluation of perceptual and cognitive processes regulating social interactions is advocated.

## INTRODUCTION

The concept of social stress finds its origin in the observation that high population densities lead to behavioural and physiological responses that are characteristic of stress. A vast amount of literature describing these responses in many different animal species, including domestic animals is available (cf. Dantzer and Raab, 1985, for a recent review). However, the precise delineation of the responsible factors, the exact nature of the response and the mechanisms leading from social factors to altered behaviour and physiology are not yet elucidated. This is unfortunate since the term social stress is normally used to refer to precise intermediate mechanisms (e.g., activation of the pituitary-adrenal axis) accounting for the effects of a set of stimuli on a given physiological function. The example of the influence of social factors on reproduction will serve to illustrate that this is far from being the case and that the concept of social stress can actually be misleading. Another limitation of the concept of social stress is that by putting too much emphasis on negative aspects of life in social groups it leads to the neglect of more positive aspects of social life such as cooperation and social support.

## SOCIAL INFLUENCES ON REPRODUCTION

In stress theory, the stress reaction is accompanied by a shut-off of all physiological functions that do not take part directly in resistance to stressors. It is the case for growth as well as reproduction. According to Selye, the mechanisms responsible for this interaction are endocrine in nature since the release of catabolic stress hormones (catecholamines and glucocorticoids) is incompatible with the release of anabolic hormones (growth hormone and gonadal hormones).

Endocrinologists have postulated that such interactions account for variations in population density. It is well known that in many species, density is far below the reproductive potential even in conditions in which environmental factors (climatic factors, food, predators, pathogens) are not limiting. In addition, some species can display drastic reductions in population size when density reaches a certain level, even if there is no shortage of resources. The usual explanation put forward for such observations is that population density is dependent on social factors. If the number of individuals in a given population is excessive, social mechanisms that normally regulate interactions between individuals and social groups are no longer effective. The increase in the number of social interactions acts as a stressor and triggers activation of the pituitary-adrenal axis. This in turn-reduces fertility and resistance to disease, which allows for a decrease in population density.

This hypothesis of a stress densostat regulating population size seems to be supported by many experimental data obtained mainly in populations of rodents allowed to reproduce in a laboratory environment with resources freely available. Under these conditions, animals display symptoms of pituitary-adrenal activation and reduced fertility. Whether the later is due to stress in the Selyan sense can be, however, disputed. There is actually little direct evidence for increased aggressive interactions in crowded populations. In addition, the decrease in the size of the population is mainly due to an increase in the frequency of deviant or abnormal sexual and maternal behaviours, as expressed by Calhoun in the concept of "behavioural sink".

According to sociobiologists, regulation of population size does not normally occur through stress mechanisms but through territoriality and emigration. Two extreme categories of species can be distinguished; opportunist species on one end, which have a high reproduction potential and of which the density is close to reproductive capacities when environmental conditions are favorable; competitive species on the other end, of which the density is well below reproductive capacities. The former species are very much dependent on environmental resources and in case of shortage of resources, extinguish or migrate. The later species are more stable and they manage to get the maximum from their ecological niche through complex social relationships requiring cooperation between group members. Within this perspective, rodents are atypical in the sense that they can use one or the other strategy, depending on the species and the resources available, whereas most species of birds and mammals that have been domesticated belong to the second category.

The potential for population growth is dependent on the sensitivity of the reproductive system to environmental factors that are predictive of the availablity of resources. This is particularly the case in seasonaly reproductive species. The efficiency of this primary regulating mechanism can be improved by social factors, as pointed out by McClintock (1981). Social signals among groups of females can either enhance or suppress ovarian cyclicity and modulate the interactions between female behavior and ovarian cycle components. Suppressive social influences on reproduction are found in many species ranging from canids to primates and ungulates. The social group can be a familial group or a harem. Reproduction is often limited to one breeding pair and other members of the group are excluded from the reproductive circuit so that they can provide help for exploiting environmental resources and care of the youngs. In callitrichids such as tamarins and marmosets, the reproductively active female inhibits by her presence ovarian cyclicity and reproduction in other females, including her daughters. Isolation of the sexually inhibited females is sufficient to restore ovarian cyclicity and sexual behavior (Abbott et al., 1988; Savage et al., 1988). Aggressive encounters between animals are unlikely to be responsible for this inhibition since there is no evidence of overt aggression and the same phenomenon can be obtained simply by exposure of females to the odor of the sexually active female. In other species, however, such as the talapoin monkey, inhibition of ovarian activity is due to aggression from the dominant female. Similar phenomena may be found in males.

Social influences on reproduction are not only inhibitory. In many instances, social factors such as the olfactory signals from a cyclic female or the stimuli emanating from a male induce estrous synchrony.

These data are important because they show that social influences on reproduction must be considered as part of an adaptive response to the environment in which the species under consideration has evolved rather than as an artefact or a manifestation of a stress response.

## SOCIAL SUPPORT

In social groups, individuals benefit from the presence of other members of the group. The concept of social facilitation which refers to the fact that a behavioral pattern is expressed at a higher frequency and/or intensity by members of a group than by individually-housed animals is a clear example of this aspect. Another related concept is social synchrony which refers to the fact that the occurrence of an activity in one animal at a given time increases the probability of occurrence of the same activity in other members of the group at the same time.

The benefit of being a member of a group is also apparent when animals are exposed to stressful situations. In general, an individual is less distressed when exposed to a stressor in presence of members of his group than when exposed alone. In an experiment representative of this type of research, pigs previously trained to obtain food by rooting a switch panel in a Skinner box were submitted to extinction (i.e., food was no longer delivered after each panel press) either individually or in pairs. Individual pigs displayed behavioural and physiological signs of frustration. The same symptoms were observed in animals exposed by pairs to the frustration situation, when pairs were formed with animals coming from different social groups, so that pair members were not previously acquainted. In this case, intense fighting developed between members of the pairs. In contrast, when two pigs from the same pen were exposed to the frustration situation, there was little or no sign of excitation (Arnone and Dantzer, 1980).

The presence or absence of social companions has therefore major effects on various physiological and behavioural responses in animals and the presence of, or interactions with these individuals appear to moderate the impact of environmental stressors. However, as proposed by Epley (1974), the mere presence of a companion is not sufficient. The first condition is that the companion remains calm in front of the threatening situation. The second condition is that the presence of the companion interferes with the subject's reactions to aversive situations.

In addition to the possible buffering effect of belongness to a social group on response to stressors, life in social groups also provides social mechanisms serving the restoration of social relationships disturbed by aggression or environmental stressors. The extent to which these conciliatory mechanisms described in monkey groups (De Waal, 1984) are also operating in domestic animals is not clear at the present time.

CONCLUSION

Our discussion of the concept of social stress has been voluntarily limited to the consideration of the shortcomings of this concept for the description and understanding of social influences on individual physiology and to the problems coming from its overemphasis on negative influences of social membership. In this discussion, we have carefully avoided to add another complex matter, represented by the concepts of territoriality and dominance which are an inherent component of the description of the effects of social factors on individuals.

To take just one example, fighting that occurs in regrouped pigs is supposed to lead to the establishment of dominance-subordination hierarchies. These hierarchies are claimed to regulate access to resources by allowing precedence to the dominant animal. Such a description implies first that the quality of the subsequent dominance order depends on the amount of fighting which occurs at regrouping and second, that the dominant animal is likely to have priority of access to the different items which must be shared with other members of the group. The implication for the concept of social stress is that this phenomenon should be unevenly distributed between members of the groups and that subordinates should be more affected than dominant animals.

We have already pointed out in a previous paper (Dantzer and Raab, 1985) that such a description is oversimplified. In the search for more relevant descriptions of the way behavioural and physiological patterns of response relate to each other in animals belonging to a same social group, the perceptual/cognitive aspects of the behavioural patterns presented by the different members of the social group should be given more emphasis. This cannot be done without a thorough description of what is happening. During an aggressive encounter for instance, it is more useful to know what pattern of agonistic behaviour is displayed (e.g., offense or defense) than to summarize the situation by its supposed outcome, i.e. the dominance order of each animal. In addition, it is necessary to understand the way social companions are perceived and classified by the individual under investigation (social cognition). Finally, in view of the data available on the importance of coping mechanisms in stress reactions, the description of the situation in terms of controllability (the way social companions' behaviour is amenable to the subject's own actions) and predictability (the extent to which the subject can predict the outcomes of his interactions with conspecifics) cannot be avoided. This is much more difficult to do than to limit oneself to a labeling of what is happening by the short hand term of social stress. It explains why the concept of social stress is still likely to lead a long and prosperous life before being rejected.

## REFERENCES

Abbott, D.M., Hodges, J.K. and George, L.M. 1988. Social status controls LH secretion and ovulation in female marmoset monkeys (Callithrix jacchus). J. Endocr., 117, 329-339.

Arnone, M. and Dantzer, R. 1980. Does frustration induce aggression in pigs? Appl. Anim. Ethol., 6, 351-362.

Dantzer, R. and Raab, A. 1985. On the interpretation and significance of behavioural and physiological indicators of stress related to social space in domestic animals. In "Social space for domestic animals" (ed. R. Zayan) (Nijhoff, Dordrecht), pp.3-14.

Epley, S.W. 1974. Reduction of the behavioral effects of aversive stimulation by the presence of companions. Psychol. Bull., 81, 271-283.

McClintock, M.K. 1981. Social control of the ovarian cycle and the function of estrous synchrony. Amer. Zool., 21, 243-256.

Savage, A., Ziegler, T.E. and Snowdon, C.T. 1988. Socio-sexual development, pair bond formation and mechanisms of fertility suppression in female Cotton-top tamarins (Sanguinus oedipus oedipus). Amer. J. Primatol., 14, 345-359.

De Waal, F.B.M. 1984. Coping with social tension: sex differences in the effect of food provision to small rhesus monkey groups. Anim. Behav., 32, 765-773.

# MECHANISMS OF COPING IN SOCIAL SITUATIONS

P.R. Wiepkema and W.G.P. Schouten

Agricultural University, Department of Animal Husbandry and
Ethology, Marijkeweg 40, 6709 PG Wageningen, The Netherlands

## ABSTRACT

Social organization relies on many and quite divergent
mechanisms; only some are discussed. Adequate organization of
adult animals is only possible when these animals had a species-
specific development including rich and unrestricted social contacts in early life. These contacts enable sociability and normal
learning capability. In the adult stage social stability is
optimal when the individuals involved know each other reliably.
High level of individual recognition implies much cognitive
effort. Social stressors reduce individual recognition and thereby
the controllability of (social) environmental changes. Social
stressors may evoke two individual bound types of coping; active
or passive coping. These types differ behaviourally and physiolo-
gically. Finally conspecifics may support each other and by this
reduce stress of a companion. Information about danger can easily
be transmitted through a whole population. Social support and
social suspicion may be important determinants of the quality of
man-animal interactions.

## INTRODUCTION

A pretty long time ago Guhl and Allee (1944) published a
paper in which they showed that removing on alternate days one hen
from an established flock and replacing this hen by a newcomer led
to disorganization of the flock and to a reduced feed intake and
egg production. Obviously social stability is an important factor
to guarantee good production in social animals. We may even go
further and state that social stability is a relevant determinant
of morbidity and mortality as suggested by the data of Weber and
Van der Walt (1973) with respect to animals in captivity or in the
wild (Bradley et al., 1980; brown antechinus). What does social
stability imply and which mechanisms are involved? We will discuss
four mechanisms or aspects that significantly determine how
individual vertebrates cope in stressful social situations. These
aspects are the following:

1. Ontogenetic processes generating sociability and learning
   capability.
2. Social interactions reflecting individual information and

8

recognition.

3. Types of behavioural and neuro-endocrine coping mechanisms.

4. Social support and suspicion.

We discuss these mechanisms from the point of view that the kind of vertebrates we are talking about (mammals, birds) basically are information processing entities (cf. Inglis, 1983). Our approach is a cognitive ethological one in which the role of the central nervous system is central and crucial.

## ONTOGENETIC MECHANISMS

Full adaptation of the adult vertebrate to its Umwelt always results from a complicated and sometimes long lasting developmental process. The essence of this process is an age specific interaction between the individual's genetic disposition and its changing internal and external environment. The first stage of this development is known under the heading of embryology. For the ethologist those stages are of great interest during which the final shaping of the central nervous system takes place (cf. Bullock, 1977). This shaping is effectuated by the interplay of specific incoming information and specific neurons active at that time and going to be connected with other neurons or specific target organs (receptors, muscle units, glands). Those elements and connections which resound first or best to this incoming information appear to be selected as the ones that survive; the others die and disappear soon (cf. Changeux, 1985).

Although in the prehatching (cf. Tschanz and Hirsbrunner-Scharf, 1975) or the prenatal (cf. vom Saal, 1983) period environmental stimuli perceived at that time may strongly influence later and even adult social behaviour, we will restrict ourselves to some utmost relevant events occurring in the period shortly after hatching or birth.

First during (early) youth interactions take place between the young animal and his/her mother, father or other conspecifics (or even non-conspecifics). These contacts determine with whom the juvenile will become to interact socially or not (for a full discussion of the processes involved see: Barnett, 1981; Bateson,

1983, 1984; Chalmers, 1983; Immelman, 1983; Marler, 1984; Slater, 1983). Some of these processes refer to filial imprinting (young-parent(s) attachment), others to sexual imprinting determining the choice of a later sexual or social partner. Interactions with humans during a critical period for imprinting may lead to a strong attachment of animals to their human caretaker (cf. Sambraus, 1975).

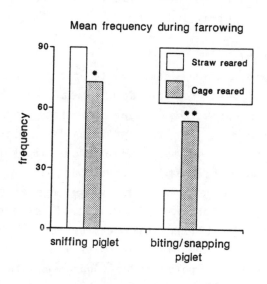

Fig. 1    Mean frequency of sniffing or biting/snapping piglets by the sow during the first 6 hours after delivery of her first piglet (first litter). The first 8 weeks of their life 6 gilts were reared in a strawpen and 6 gilts grew up in a farrowing crate without straw. From week 9 on all gilts were kept in strawpens.
    * P < 0.1; ** P < 0.005 . $\chi^2$ test (from Schouten, 1986).

The available evidence unambiguously leads to the conclusion, that in social species the individuals involved should exercise a given amount of social interaction (play-like behaviour) during a critical period in order to behave much later in a species-specific way towards congeners. If such an exercise did not take place, for instance, when reared in isolation or kept in a setting that did not allow normal play behaviour, permanent and sometimes dramatic abberations in social behaviour may occur (fig. 1) (Broom, 1982; Hemsworth et al, 1977; Kruijt, 1964; Schouten, 1986;

Wiepkema, 1987). Therefore sociability being the capability to behave socially in an adequate way depends on satisfactory ontogenetic conditions.

In all those husbandry systems where we keep farm animals in groups, we should have or obtain excellent knowledge of the ontogenetic conditions required for normal social behaviour.

A second and quite general characteristic of vertebrates is their capability to detect and to store sequential (causal) relationships in their Umwelt (Dickinson, 1980). By this we mean that animals like farm animals are able to discover that the probability of a given event ($E_2$) depends on the occurrence of a preceding event ($E_1$). In formula this is the case when:

$$P_{E_2/E_1} \neq P_{E_2/no-E_1}$$

$E_1$ may represent an operant (e.g. manipulating a nipple) evoking $E_2$ (e.g. availability of water) or $E_1$ may be an external event (e.g. specific sounds) that signals $E_2$ (e.g. arrival of the caretaker): both types of learning are described as operant learning and conditioning respectively. Such relationships are often described as contingencies in the environment or conditional events.

Operant learning brings about controllability (implying predictability) of environmental changes, while conditioning implies predictability only. As we shall see later both terms controllability and predictability are of crucial importance in evaluating stress.

Contrary to what might be expected the available evidence suggests, that the ability to practice operant learning, that is to control environmental changes, does not arise automatically. This ability strongly depends on early experiences. For instance, infant monkeys raised with an artificial mother and having no contact with age mates show severe learning deficits. Such monkeys are no more interested in Umwelt changes and behave apathetically (Mason, 1978). Experiencing a non-reactive mother may lead to the infant's conviction that its behaviour does not have consequences. Such a belief will later on seriously handicap this animal in learning situations and especially in those which are typical for social interactions. We do not know in how far the lack of early experience in learning - as described just before - may disturb learning capabilities permanently.

We have, however, to take into account the possibility that shortcomings in early learning experience may strongly hamper adult social contacts which require a high learning capability.

In sum: in early life processes take place that in social animals determine their sociability and presumably their learning capabilities. Both mechanisms are of great importance for the realization and maintenance of social systems characterized by a minimum of stress.

SOCIAL INFORMATION AND RECOGNITION

Social situations are present when the behaviour of (mostly) conspecifics is interdependent. Such is the case when the individuals in question forage or rest together, move in company, form reproductive units, keep a non-random mutual distance, etc. This interdependence of behaviour has been based on the ability of many organisms to develop and maintain a so called social organization.

It is not our intention to describe, let alone to discuss, the rich diversity of social organizations realized in the animal kingdom. In vertebrates this may vary from temporary units for reproduction in which individual recognition is presumably low (for instance, sticklebacks), to large swarms or schools that move and rest together (for instance, starlings out of the season), to groups of conspecifics that form permanent societies in which complex interindividual relationships originate and are maintained. In the following we will focus on groups formed by some dozens of conspecifics in which a high level of individual recognition may exist; this is the basic group size of most if not all wild ancestors of our present day farm animals. The existence of supergroups of (ten) thousands of animals in modern husbandry will be discussed separately.

No doubt all the different types of social organization have their own survival value in terms of being adapted to a specific ecological niche. Nevertheless these social organizations are not without their pros and cons (Huntingford, 1984). Pros include the facilitation of finding food and water, a mutual support in defense situations and enhanced thermoregulatory capabilities. To the cons belong the intensified competition for scarce commodities and the heavy cognitive efforts.

What do we mean with the expression cognitive efforts? If we take organisms like mammals and birds basically as information processing entities, then this refers to their well testified trait to actively gather, store and implement information in an adaptive way. Exploratory behaviour and its impact on later actions of the animal form an excellent illustration of the processes we have in mind now (cf. Archer and Birke, 1983). When put in a not too strange environment an animal will first start to explore the physical and spatial characteristics of that environment before making contact with eventual conspecifics (fig. 2) (Colpaert and Wiepkema, 1976). This exploration leads to the formation of a so called cognitive map (Morris, 1983; Toates, 1986; Tolman, 1948) to be used, for instance, when the organism forages, rests or behaves socially.

Cognitive effort stands for the amount and quality of information the organism collects and processes to make up an adequate and reliable neural representation of its environment. The more complex the subject's environment the heavier the cognitive effort to form such a neural blue-print. In social animals conspecifics (and sometimes non-conspecifics) are not only inherent parts of their Umwelt, but also the most dynamic and complex ones. There is abundant evidence that at least in mammals and birds social conspecifics recognize each other in much detail (Beer, 1975; Stoddart, 1980; Walther, 1984). This recognition may vary from identifying another organism as some conspecific, or a group member, to recognizing it as a particular individual. In the latter case we speak of individual recognition. Clearly this range of recognition is one of increasing complexity and thus one of increasing cognitive effort.

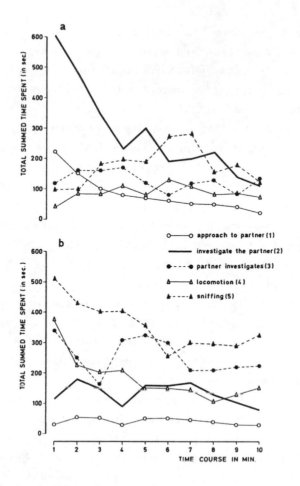

Fig. 2. Time course of 5 exploratory behaviours of 2 male rats (17 pairs) brought together in the same cage. Male a (upper graph) had been placed into the cage 10 min. prior to male b (lower graph). After Colpaert and Wiepkema, 1976.

Individual recognition is evidenced when the behaviour of a given individual depends predictably on the behaviour or presence of at least one other and particular group member; a so called specific dyadic relationship. When individual recognition is present this may again hold different levels of complexity. First in a group one individual may recognize only one or some members of his group individually, the others being only interchangeable group members. Second, the information an individual has about another one may be superficial or very detailed and flexible.

Third, an organism may not only be acquainted with most if not all other members of the group individually, it also may be informed about individual relationships existing between these other members of the group. No doubt, the latter information is the most complex one: it certainly exists in humans, and has been shown in some infra-human primates (De Waal, 1982). We cannot exclude that spurs of this type of individual recognition may also exist in pigs, horses and cattle. This point needs urgently systematic investigation, since it pertains to the question how group size and composition in farm animals can be optimized.

The conclusion from the foregoing is that in social groups a highly important coping mechanism is represented by the capability to collect, to store and to use information about general and specific qualities of group members. This information enables a social individual to anticipate or to control conspecific's behaviour. A good illustration hereof is the frequently analyzed phenomenon of dominance relationships reflecting the finding, that in specific dyads one individual consistently dominates and the other gives way. The phrase "consistent" is not identical to permanent: over time dominance relationships may change as a result of natural changes in group composition. For a broader discussion of the concept of dominance see Bernstein (1981).

Individual recognition includes two aspects:
a. differentiation of the other individual on the basis of visual, auditory, smell and other characteristics and
b. correlating these characteristics with the specific behaviour patterns of that same individual.
This latter aspect does not only comprise knowledge of the routines of that other animal, but also information about how this other animal may interfere with own behaviour. Especially this latter point implies a quite complicated knowledge, since the functional role of any other individual may also depend on time (day, season, oestrus cycles, etc.) and space (feeding site, resting site, strange area, etc.).

The great benefit of all this knowledge is that in a well integrated group individuals may reliably predict and control each others behaviour. This predictability/controllability is disturbed and reduced by social stressors that bring about stress of the individuals involved; stress itself becoming visible and measurable in terms of conflict or disturbed behaviour, emotional expressions and a specific pattern of neuroendocrine changes (Bohus et al. 1987; Dantzer and Morméde, 1983; Simonov, 1986; Wiepkema, 1987).

Some examples of social stressors are the following events or situations. First the introduction of strange individuals to a well-established group or the removal of core members of such a group immediately reduces the reliability of existing social relationships. A similar situation is present when a totally new group is formed. In this context it is interesting and useful for practical husbandry to know whether relationships between conpecifics brought together in the (sub)adult phase may develop a same quality (stability) as those stemming from early life interactions

A second potential stressor is group size. The larger the group the smaller the possibility and the capability to become acquainted with each group member individually. This implies encounters with potential strangers and a reduction of predictability/controllability. In fact we know little to nothing of how members of a supergroup (thousands of members) regulate their social relationships. The answer may be the formation of many subgroups, or starting to interact as neutral conspecifics as may occur in natural swarms and schools. We have to be better informed about what happens in the supergroups (hens, pigs, cattle) existing in modern husbandry.

A third stressor is scarcity or even absence of relevant environmental features (food, nesting sites, opportunity to perform specific behaviour like rooting, scratching, dust bathing and others). Under such conditions confinement may evoke severe social frictions and lead to the occurrence of injurious behaviour. Under natural conditions such stressors would immediately stimulate (adaptive) dispersion.

In sum: a second and utmost relevant coping mechanism in social situations is the capability to recognize conspecifics even at the individual level (a first class cognitive performance!). By this, control of the social environment becomes optimal.

TYPES OF BEHAVIOURAL AND NEUROENDOCRINE MECHANISMS.

From the foregoing it will be clear that we consider the phenomenon of stress as a response state of the individual resulting from a reduced controllability and/or predictability of relevant Umwelt changes. Formulated this way stress always reflects an existing and significant information deficit; it is thereby basically (also) a cognitive problem.

By definition cognition is localized in the central nervous system. Although it is clear that integrated physiological and behavioural events need the participation of the whole brain it is becoming clear that different areas of the brain have their own and specific contribution to these integrated events. In the stress response a crucial role is for the hippocampus and the amygdala-hypothalamus complex, all being parts of the so called limbic system. (Smelik, 1987; Warburton, 1987; Wiepkema et al. 1980). While one of the functions of the hippocampus appears to be to match incoming information with the already existing one, parts of the amygdala control the performance of motivationally adequate behaviours; finally the hypothalamus realizes a critical connection between the neural and endocrine systems.

As expected there is a different neuroendocrine response between winners and loosers, or dominants and subordinates, or those individuals that control their environment and those who only can predict environmental changes. Such a difference has been indicated by Henry (1976), who proposed that the first group of animals performs a predominantly sympathetic response (increase of (nor)adrenaline plasma levels, no definite change in corticosteroid levels and an increased testosterone level), while the second group - the loosers - show a rise in the pituitary - adrenocortical response (increased ACTH and corticosteroid plasma levels, no change in catecholamines and a decrease of testosterone); all these changes have a long term character. In this context it is intruiging to notice the richness of corticoid receptors in the brain (cf. McEwen, 1987).

TABEL 1    Individual characteristics of active and passive
copers (rats); after Bohus et al. 1987.

| active | | passive |
| --- | --- | --- |
| defensive, escape | aggressive behaviour against dominant | freezing |
| | spatial orientation | |
| many errors | 1) changing intramaze configuration | few errors |
| few errors | 2) changing extramaze beacons | many errors |
| high | blood pressure reactivity | low |
| tachycardia | cardiac reactivity | bradycardia |
| high | (nor) adrenaline reactivity | low |
| high | corticosterone reactivity | low |

The surprising point we want to emphasize now is that in
(social) stress conditions two types of individuals may emerge
(cf. table 1): those who cope in an active way and those who do so
in a more passive way (Bohus et al. 1987; von Holst, 1986; Koolhaas et al. 1986). Short term reactions of the so called active
copers are predominantly sympathetic and characterized by an
increased blood pressure, a high reactivity of catecholamines and
corticosteroids, performance of offensive or escape behaviour, and
a strong tendency to develop routines). The passive copers show a
predominantly parasympathetic way of reacting; for instance, a
decrease of blood pressure, a low reactivity of catecholamines
and corticosteroids, performance of freezing behaviour and a weak
development of routines. Comparable types of coping have been
described for dogs (Corson and Corson, 1976); such a distinction
may also underlay the large individual differences with respect to
performing, for instance, stereotypies as described for veal
calves (Wiepkema et al. 1987). Recently Koolhaas et al. (1987)
also reported for both type of copers a different response of the
immune system to social stressors.

    The adaptive significance of both types of coping is presum-
ably related to fluctuations in population density occurring under

natural conditions. Van Oortmerssen et al. (1985) presented good evidence that during crowding the passive copers disperse and, moreover, that this type of animals has better capabilities to survive in a new environment than the active copers. A dramatic increase of morbidity and mortality resulting from severe, but natural social stressors has been described for the brown antechinus (Bradley et al. 1980).

In sum: a third and most complex coping mechanism during social stress is represented by the neuroendocrine response especially since individuals may differentiate into two types of copers; the active and the passive ones. This differentiation may also be present in farm animals; systematic research on this point is urgently needed.

SOCIAL SUPPORT AND SUSPICION.

One of the most intriguing findings in the research of von Holst (1986) on social stress in Tupayas is that joining a male and a female sometimes may lead to severe fights in such a way that one of the individuals will die; however, in other cases nearly immediately an harmonious pair originates. In these latter pairs a strong reduction of adrenocortical activity and a significant decrease of heart beat frequency were recorded. Harmonious fitting of two animals resulted in a remarkable reduction of well-known stress parameters. Presumably such an effect also reduces morbidity of both animals (von Holst, 1986; 1987). This finding demonstrates an important and positive effect of what could be called social support. A comparable phenomenon might have been described by Arnone and Dantzer (1980), when they found that the presence of a well-known congener reduced a typical stress response in pigs when being frustrated. It is certainly not too far sought to mention in this context the research of Nerem et al. (1980), who discovered that handling rabbits in a friendly way significantly reduced the development of atherosclerosis.

Social support of animals, even when given by familiar humans, may substantially reduce their stress symptoms. In fact much of the work of Hemsworth and coworkers on animal-men interactions may be explained in this way (Gonyou et al. 1986; Hemsworth et al. 1986; 1987).

Returning to the data of von Holst, we have to add the puzzling question why some pairs of Tupayas fit immediately and others do not and, may be, never. We had a comparable experience when joining an estrous female with an adult male (mice, rats). Some combinations were immediately successful (i.e. occurrence of copulations), while other combinations did not work. As yet we have no explanation for these differences. It might be, however, that if something like social support exists in a given species, not all combinations are equally successful (apart from some self-evident examples of mutual rivalry of, for instance, adult males). On this point systematic research on social groups of farm animals is urgently needed.

If social support exists, one also may expect social suspicion. Some animals may not fit each other and for some good reason may even distrust each other. Henceforth they may avoid each other where possible. Little to nothing is known on this point. However, some interesting data are available about such relationships towards non-conspecifics.

Lorenz (1952) was one of the first who hinted this possibility in his famous research on jackdaws. Adult birds teach naive ones to avoid certain non-conspecific configurations (cat, predator, black cloth, etc.). Recently Curio et al. (1978) showed in an as simple as elegant experiment, that in black birds mobbing behaviour serves the transmission of enemy recognition through a population of blackbirds.

In this analysis it was not only found that even false information could be transmitted, but also that several birds may successively be involved in this transmission. This investigation illustrates a mechanism, that may play an important role in groups of farm animals with respect to their evaluation of human caretakers. In order to trust or to distrust humans it is not necessary, that each individual animal in a stall has contacted a human being regularly or intensively. For instance, in a stall with pigs negative experience of only some individuals with human beings may suffice to be signalled through the whole stall, making most if not all other pigs suspicious or afraid of human beings. It is

clear that such a cultural transmission of "danger information"
has great adaptive value. In present day husbandry systems this
type of information - trust or distrust of humans - may be a
factor of great significance in determining the quality of man-
animal interactions involved and thus of the social stability of
these groups.

In sum: a fourth coping mechanism in social situations implies the capability to support each other and by this reducing
stress. Closely related with this characteristic  is the capability to inform each other about potential danger. Both mechanisms are
typical cognitive designs relevant in social situations.

REFERENCES
Archer, J. and Birke, L. (Eds). 1983. Exploration in animals and
     humans. Van Nostrand Reinhold, U.K.
Arnone, M. and Dantzer, R. 1980. Does frustration induce aggres-
     sion in pigs. Appl. Anim. Ethol., 6, 351-362.
Barnett, S.A. 1981. Modern Ethology. Oxford Univ. Press, Oxford.
Bateson, P.G. 1983. Genes, environment and the development of
     behaviour. In: "Animal Behaviour". (Eds. T.R. Halliday and
     P.J.B. Slater) (Blackwell, Oxford). pp. 52-81.
Bateson, P.G. 1984. Genes, evolution, and learning. In "The biolo-
     gy of learning" (Eds. P. Marler and H.S. Terrace) (Springer,
     Berlin). pp. 75-88.
Beer, G.C. 1975. Multiple functions and gull displays. In "Func-
     tion and Evolution in Behaviour" (Eds. G. Baerends, C. Beer
     and A. Manning). (Clarendon Press, Oxford). pp. 16-54.
Bernstein, L.S., 1981. Dominance: the baby and the bathwater. The
     behavioural and brain sciences, 4, 419-457.
Bohus, B. Benus, R.F., Fokkema, D.S., Koolhaas, J.M., Nyakas, C.,
     Van Oortmerssen, G.A., Prins, A.J.A., De Ruiter, A.J.H.,
     Scheurink A.J.W. and Steffens, A.B. 1987. Neuroendocrine
     states and behavioural and physiological stress responses. In
     "Neuropeptides and brain function" (Eds. E.R. de Kloet, V.M.
     Wiegant and D. de Wied). Progr. Brain Research, 72, 57-70.
Bradley, A.J., McDonald, I.R. and Lee, A.K,. 1980. Stress and
     mortality in a small marsupial (Antechinus stuartii,
     MacLeay). Gen. comp. endocrinol., 40, 188-200.
Broom, D.M., 1982. Husbandry methods leading to inadequate social
     and maternal behaviour in cattle. In "Disturbed behaviour in
     farm animals" (Ed. W. Bessei) (Eugen Ulmer, Stuttgart). pp.
     42-50.
Bullock, T.H. 1977. Introduction to nervous systems. Freeman, San
     Francisco.
Changeux, J.P. 1985. Neuronal man. The biology of mind. Oxford
     Univ. Press. Oxford.
Chalmers, N. 1983. The development of social relationship. In
     "Animal Behaviour 3" (Eds. T.R. Halliday and P.J.B. Slater)
     (Blackwell, Oxford). pp. 114-148.

Corson, S.A. and Corson, E.O.L. 1976. Constitutional differences in physiological adaptation to stress and distress. In "Psychopathology of human adaptation" (Ed. G. Serban) (Plenum Press, New York). pp. 77-94.

Colpaert, F.C. and Wiepkema, P.R. 1976. Effects of ventromedial hypothalamic lesions on spontaneous intraspecies aggression in male rats. Behav. Biol., 16, 117-125.

Curio, E., Ernst K. and Vieth, W. 1978. Cultural transimission of enemy recognition: one fuction of mobbing. Science, 202, 899-901.

Dantzer, R. and Mormède, P. 1985. Stress in farm animals: a need for reëvaluation. J. anim. Sci., 57, 6-18.

Dickinson, A. 1980. Contemporary animal learning theory. Cambridge Univer. Press., Cambridge.

Gonyou, H.W., Hemsworth, P.H. and Barnett, J.L. 1986. Effects of frequent interaction with humans on growing pigs. Appl. Anim. Behav. Sci., 16, 269-278.

Gould, J.L. and Marler, P. 1987. Learning by instinct. Scientific American, 256, 62-73.

Gull, A.M. and Allee, W.C. 1944. Some measurable effects of social organization in flocks of hens. Physiol. Zool., 17, 320-347.

Hemsworth, P.H. Barnett, J.L. and Hansen, C. 1987. The influence of inconsistent handling by humans on the behaviour, growth and corticosteroids of young pigs. Appl. Anim. Behav. Sci., 17, 245-252.

Hemsworth, P.H. Beilharz, R.G. and Galloway D.B., 1977. Influence of social conditions during rearing on the sexual behaviour of the domestic boar. Anim. Prod., 24, 245-251.

Henry, J.P. 1976. Mechanisms of psychosomatic disease in animals. Adv. Vet. Sci. Comp. Med., 20, 115-145.

Holst, D. von, 1986. Vegetative and somatic components of tree shrews'behaviour. J. auton. nerv. syst. Suppl., 657-670.

Holst, D. von, 1987. Sozialer Stress bei Tier und Mensch. In "Vorträge zum Thema Mensch und Tier. Band V" (Eds M. Röhrs und H. Meyer). (Schafer, Hannover). pp. 27-51.

Huntingford, F. 1984. The study of animal behaviour. Chapman and Hall, Londen.

Immelman, K. 1984. The natural history of bird learning. In "The biology of learning" (Eds. P. Marler and H.S. Terrace) (Springer, Berlin). pp. 271-288.

Inglis, I.R. 1983. Towards a cognitive theory of exploratory behaviour. In "Exploration in animals and humans". (Eds. J. Archer and L. Birke) (van Nostrand Reinhold, U.K.). pp. 72-116.

Koolhaas, J.M., Fokkema, D.S., Bohus, B., and Oortmerssen, G.A. van. 1986. Individual differentiation in blood pressure reactivity and behaviour of male rats. In "Biobehavioural Bases of coronary heart disease. Vol 3" (Eds. T.M. Dembroski, T.H. Schmidt, and G. Blümchen) (Karger, Basel). pp. 517-526.

Koolhaas, J.M., Heynen, C.J., Ballieux, R.E. and Bohus, B. 1987. Social structure, psychological stress and immunity. Proc. 28th Dutch. Federation Meeting. P. 265.

Kruyt, J.P. 1964. Ontogeny of social behaviour in Burmese Red Junglefawl. Behaviour, Suppp. XII, 1-201.

Lorenz, K. 1952. King Solomon's Ring. Methuen, London.

Marler, P. 1984. Song learning: innate species differences in the learning process. In "The biology of learning" (Eds. P. Marler and H.S. Terrace) (Springer, Berlin). pp. 289-309.

Mason, W.A. 1978. Social experience and primate cognitive development . In "The development of behavior (Eds. G.M. Burghardt and M. Bekoff) (Garland, New York). pp. 233-251.

McEwen, B.S. and Brinton, R.E. 1987. Neuroendocrine aspects of adaptation. In "Neuropeptides and brain functions" (Eds. E.R. de Kloet, V.M. Wiegant and D. de Wied). Prog. Brain Res., $72$, 11-26.

Morris, R.G.M. 1983. Neural subsystems of exploration in rats. In "Exploration in animals and humans" (Eds. J. Archer and L. Birke) (Van Nostrand Reinhold, U.K.). pp. 117-146.

Nerem, R.M., Levesque, M.J. and Cornhill, J.F. 1980. Social environment as a factor in diet-induced atherosclerosis. Science, $208$, 1475-1476.

Oliverio, A. 1987. Endocrine aspects of stress: central and peripheral mechanisms. In "Biology of stress in farm animals: an integrative approach" (Eds. P.R. Wiepkema and P.W.M. van Adrichem) (Nijhoff, Dordrecht). pp. 3-12.

Van Oortmerssen, G.A., Benus, L. and Dijk, D.J. 1985. Studies in wild house mice: genotype-environment interactions for attach latency. Nethl. J. Zool., $35$, 155-169.

Saal, F.S. vom. 1983. The interaction of circulating oestrogens and androgens in regulating mammalian sexual differentation. In "Hormones and behaviour in higher Vertebrates" (Eds. J. Balthazart, E. Pröve and R. Gilles) (Springer, Berlin). pp. 159-177.

Sambraus, H.H. and Sambraus, D. 1975. Prägung von Nutztieren auf Menschen. Z. Tierpsychol., $38$, 1-17.

Schouten, W.G.P. 1986. Rearing conditions and behaviour in pigs. Ph.D. Thesis. Agricultural Univ. Wageningen.

Smelik, P.G. 1987. Adaptation and brain function. In "Neuropeptides and brain function" (Eds. E.R. de Kloet, V.M. Wiegant and D. de Wied). Prog. Brain Res., $72$, 3-9.

Simonov, G.P.V., 1986. The emotional brain. Plenum Press, New York.

Slater, P.J.B. 1983. The development of individual behaviour. In "Animal behaviour 3" (Eds. T.R. Halliday and P.J.B. Slater) (Blackwell, Oxford). pp. 82-113.

Stoddart, D.M. 1980. The ecology of vertebrate olfaction. Chapman and Hall, London.

Toates, F.M. 1983. Exploration as a motivational and learning system: a cognitive incentive view. In "Exploration in animals and humans" (Eds. J. Archer and L. Birke) (van Nostrand Reinhold, U.K.). pp. 55-71.

Toates, F. 1986. Motivational systems. Cambridge Univ. Press. Cambridge.

Tolman, E.C. 1948. Cognitive maps in rats and men. Psychol. Rev. $55$, 189-208.

Tschanz, B. and Hirsbrunner-Scharf, M. 1975. Adaptations to colony life on cliff edges: a comparative study of guillemot and razorbill chicks. In "Function and Evolution in Behaviour" (Eds. G. Baerends, C. Beer and A. Manning) (Clarendon, Oxford). pp. 358-380.

Waal, F.B.M. de. 1982. Chimpanzee politics: power and sex among apes. Jonathan Cape, London.

Walther, F.R. 1984. Communication and expression in hoofed animals. Indiana Univ. Press, Bloomington.

Warburton, D.M. 1987. The neuropsychology of stress response control. In "Biology of stress in farm animals: an integrative approach" (Eds. P.R. Wiepkema and P.W.M. van Adrichem) (Nijhoff, Dordrecht). pp. 87-100.

Weber, H.W. and Van der Walt, J.J. 1973. Cardiomyopathy in crowded rabbits. A. preliminary report. S.A. Med. J., 47, 1591-1595.

Wiepkema, P.R. 1987a. Behavioural aspects of stress. In "Biology of stress in farm animals: an integrative approach" (Eds. P.R. Wiepkema and P.W.M. van Adrichem) (Nijhoff, Dordrecht). pp. 113-133.

Wiepkema, P.R. 1987b. Development aspects of motivated behaviour in domestic animals. J. Anim. Sci., 65, 1220-1227.

Wiepkema, P.R. Van Hellemond, K.K., Roessingh, P. and Romberg, H. 1987. Behaviour and abomasal damage in individual veal calves. Appl. Anim. Behav. Sci., 18, 257-268.

Wiepkema, P.R., Koolhaas, J.M. and Olivier-Aardema, R. 1980. Adaptive aspects of neuronal elements in agonistic behaviour. Prog. Brain. Res., 53, 369-384.

# SOCIAL CONTACT REQUIREMENTS OF
# DOMESTIC PIGS ASSESSED BY BEHAVIORAL
# DEMAND FUNCTIONS

J. Ladewig and L. Matthews

Institute of Animal Husbandry and Animal Behavior
Federal Research Center of Agriculture
Trenthorst, 2061 Westerau, FRG

ABSTRACT

A method is presented by which the requirements of
various environmental stimuli can be measured quantitatively
in domestic pigs. The principle of the method is derived from
economics. Economists observe that, for some goods, the total
quantity purchased is relatively independent of increases in
price (inelastic demand). For other goods, consumption
decreases following similar price increases (elastic demand).
Commodities which are recognized as necessities show
inelastic demand, and less important items are characterized
by more elastic demand. Therefore, quantitative indices of
importance of various commodities can be derived by measuring
the slopes of the demand curves (quantity purchased as a
function of price).

The operant conditioning technique was used to generate
demand curves for different 'commodities' with domestic pigs
as 'consumers'. The pigs were trained to operate a nose plate
and social contact (door opening for 20 sec allowing nose-to-
nose contact with a familiar pig through a grill) or food
(27 g concentrate) were used as reinforcers. Reinforcement
was delivered on a fixed ratio (FR). To simulate price
increases, FR-values were increased in sequence (FR 1, 2, 5,
15, 20 and 30). Each pig was tested daily in two-hour
sessions.

Comparison of the slopes of the demand curves showed
that the requirement for social contact (slope -.5) was more
elastic than the requirement for food (slope 0). As expected,
food appeared more important than social contact. Apart from
demonstrating the relative importance of social contact and
food, the results show that it is possible to measure
requirements for a number of stimuli (such as straw and
locomotion, which is being tested in an ongoing study). Thus,
the importance of various environmental features can be
ranked quantitatively in relation to each other, so that
recommendations can be given as to which features must be
present in a housing system for domestic pigs.

INTRODUCTION

Social contact is an important aspect of life, especially for herd animals such as domestic pigs. The actual value of social contact, however, compared to other features of the environment is, for various reasons, difficult to assess. First, it seems reasonable to assume that the requirement for conspecifics varies, and that it is higher in some situations (e.g. during feeding, sleeping or investigation of new areas) than in others (e.g. during birth). Secondly, for domestic animals kept in intensive housing systems, it is reasonable to assume that social requirement depends, at least partially, upon the presence or absence of other environmental features. For instance, pigs kept without straw may have a bigger need for social contact than pigs kept on straw. And finally, the type of contact (i.e. visual, auditory, olfactory or tactile) is a confounding factor that must be taken into consideration when social requirements are considered.

In an attempt to assess quantitatively social contact requirements in pigs, a study was done using an operant conditioning procedure. The principle for the technique is derived from economics. Economists observe that, for some goods, the total quantity purchased is relatively independent of increases in price (so called inelastic demand). For other goods, consumption decreases following similar price increases (elastic demand). Commodities which are recognised as necessities show inelastic demand and less important items are characterised by more elastic demand. Therefore, a quantitative index of importance of various commodities can be calculated by measuring the slopes of the demand curves (quantity purchased as a function of price).

To generate similar demand curves using pigs as 'consumers', different 'commodities' (such as social contact or food) are presented after the pigs have paid a certain 'price' or performed a certain amount of work. The pigs are trained to operate a nose plate. In the beginning, the price

is kept low; that is, each pig has to press the nose plate
only once to obtain a certain amount of reward (e.g. 25 g
food). The ratio nose plate reactions - rewards is kept
constant or fixed; that is, the animal is tested on a fixed
ratio 1 (FR 1). Later, the FR value is increased (FR 2, 5,
10, etc.), meaning that the pig must press 2, 5, 10, etc.
times to obtain the same amount of reward.

In the present study, 4 pigs were tested for their
requirement for social contact. Outside the test situation,
they were kept in individual confinement with no visual or
tactile contact with neighboring animals. Each pig was tested
daily, 7 days a week, over a 2 h period in a special test
box. After nose plate activation, a door was automatically
opened for 20 sec. On the other side of the door, another
pig, which was familiar to the test pig, was kept. Through a
grill the two pigs were able to interact with nose-to-nose
contact.

The same 4 pigs were also tested for their food
requirements. Two of the pigs were tested first for food,
then for social contact, and the remaining two pigs were
tested first for social contact, then for food. As a control
situation, all 4 pigs were tested for door opening alone,
i.e. with no pig present on the other side of the door.
Each pig was tested for a minimum of 7 days on each FR-value,
and the results of the last 5 days were used to establish the
points in the demand curves. The pigs were tested, first, in
an ascending sequence of FR schedules and immediately
afterwards, a couple of the FR-values were repeated in a
descending sequence. The pigs were tested in a closed box,
and delivery of reinforcements plus registration of reactions
and reinforcements were handled by a special computer
program.

The result of this first study showed that the
requirement for food is inelastic, i.e. that the pigs
consumed the same amount of food independent of how hard they
had to work for it. In contrast, the requirement for social

contact is elastic, i.e. as the work load increased, relatively less contact was purchased. Quantitatively, the slope of the demand curve for food was 0, for social contact - 0.5.

As mentioned before, a control test was done with all 4 pigs, in which the requirement for door opening alone was analysed. The slope of this demand curve was - 0.6, i.e. almost as high as for social contact. We interpret this result as follows: At the time of testing, the animals had been kept in a very sterile and boring environment for over 6 months, so that even the slightest 'entertainment' (such as door opening alone) was rewarding to the animals.

The advantage of this method compared to other attempts at measuring requirements quantitatively (choice tests, maze tests etc.) are several. Firstly, the absolute amount of reward obtained has no influence on the slope of the demand curve. A similar result was found in guinea pigs that were allowed either 10 or 20 sec access to water as reinforcement (Hirsch and Collier, 1974 a, b). This result is in strong contrast to the results of a study on light requirements in chicken by Savory and Duncan (1982). If the duration of the light reward was relatively short (1 or 3 min) the animals appeared to have less light requirement than if the light was turned on for 50 min per reward. Therefore, these results did not allow any conclusions as far as light requirement in chickens are concerned.

Secondly, not only does the amount of reward have no influence on the slope of the demand curves, but also the individual demand for the reward has no influence. Thus, rats that were tested for food requirement after 22 h starvation showed demand curves with a similar slope as rats that were tested after 16 h starvation (Lea and Roper, 1977).

Thirdly, the greatest advantage of the method is, however, that it is possible to test the requirements for stimuli that appears to have nothing with each other to do. In a study on rats, reinforcement consisted of either food or electric brain stimulation at two different intensities. If this study has been conducted with only a low FR-value, one would have concluded that intensive brain stimulation was most attractive. Testing on several FR-values and calculation of slopes, however, revealed the opposite result, that food is more important than brain stimulation, independent of stimulus intensity (Hursh and Natelson, 1981).

For our work with domestic pigs it means that it is possible to isolate various environmental features and analyse the requirements for each feature under controlled conditions. Right now, we are starting a new series of tests in which the demand for locomotion or straw is studied. In the test for locomotion requirement, the pig is placed on a treadmill and reinforcement consists of 15 sec activation of the treadmill. In the test for straw requirement, activation of the nose plate results in the test chamber being moved over to a neighboring area where straw is available. After a certain amount of time, the test chamber rolls back again, forcing the pig to leave the straw.

The long term objective of these studies is to obtain a requirement index (i.e. a slope value) for as many environmental stimuli as possible, and to rank these indices on a scale. In this way, it will be possible to identify environmental stimuli (or features) that are absolutely necessary in a housing system (top portion of the scale), features that are unimportant (bottom part of scale), and a midsection that, for animal welfare reasons, must be considered when designing new housing systems.

The interpretation of the importance of these 'in between' features will, of course, depend on subjective (i.e. human) considerations. Nevertheless, establishment of the requirement indices is bound to help such considerations. Moreover, as mentioned in the beginning, the requirement for one feature (e.g. social contact) may depend partly on the presence of other features (e.g. straw) which, of course, also can be measured quantitatively with the present method.

Similarly, type and intensity of social contact can also be tested quantitatively, i.e. whether it is enough that the animals can see each other, whether nose-to-nose contact will satisfy the pigs, or whether more intimate contact is preferred.

ACKNOWLEDGEMENT

Part of the research was supported by the Alexander von Humboldt Foundation.

REFERENCES

Hirsch, E. and Collier, G. 1974 a. The ecological
    determinants of reinforcement in the guinea pig.
    Physiol. Behav. 12, 239-249.
Hirsch, E. and Collier, G. 1974 b. Effort as a determinant of
    intake and patterns of drinking in the guinea pig.
    Physiol. Behav. 12, 647-655.
Hursh, S. R. and Natelson, B. H. 1981. Electrical brain
    stimulation and food reinforcement dissociated by demand
    elasticity. Physiol. Behav. 26, 509-515.
Lea, S. E. G. and Roper, T. J. 1977. Demand for food on
    fixed-ratio schedules as a function of the quality of
    concurrently available reinforcement. J. Expl. Anal.
    Behav. 27 371-380.
Savory, C. J. and Duncan, I. J. H. 1982. Voluntary regulation
    of lighting by domestic fowl in Skinner boxes. Appl.
    Anim. Ethol. 9, 73-81.

PERSPECTIVES IN THE STUDY OF SOCIAL STRESS

R. ZAYAN
Unité de Psychobiologie
1, Place Croix du Sud
B- 1348 Louvain-la-Neuve (Belgium)

ABSTRACT

Some of the problems raised by the study of social stress in domestic animals are first discussed. These problems relate to definitions of stress, to the search of specific social stressors, to exaggerated reference being made to aggression and to agonistic status, and to hormonal responses indicating various processes other than social stress. An integrative view, taking the various levels at which social stress occurs, is outlined. Finally, the results of an experiment with laying hens are briefly summarized. They show how various indicators (behavioural, hormonal, morphological) of social stress altogether differ when birds are caged in pairs and when they are caged in triads, suggesting that the group condition increases stress.

INTRODUCTION

Once a theoretical nightmare, the concept of stress has recently been considerably clarified and has become a fruitful perspective for studying animal welfare (Wiepkema and Van Adrichem, 1987). Many pitfalls, however, remain to be avoided in the study of social stress. Some are semantic, and concern the stimuli and the responses which would be (and should be) specific of social stress. Some other are methodological; they concern some of the defects typical of many classical experiments on social stress, particularly in domestic fowl, as well as some of the problems raised by the interpretation of hormonal responses activated both by the onset of aggression and by experiences considered to be stressful. The paper will review some of these difficulties, before it attempts to describe the

31

complexity of a process such as social stress by pointing to the various levels at which it can be investigated. Because of this complexity, experiments on social stress had better be conducted with an integrative view relating the sociological aspects of stress to its mechanisms at the organic level, via the behavioural and the cognitive components of social interactions. Finally, an experiment with laying hens housed in battery cages will serve to illustrate how density may affect various indicators of stress, ranging from agonistic behaviour to adrenocortical responses.

## Conceptual problems

Because the notion of stress is not precisely a paragon of semantic clarity, it is often believed that the concept will become less vague if defined in terms of "stressors" inducing "stress responses". Thus, a range of adverse stimuli are identified as stressors (e.g. climatic, nutritional) and a range of organic responses, usually physiological ones, are taken as consistent indicators of stress (e.g. adrenomedullary or adrenocortical activity). So, at first sight the specific concept of social stress would make it possible to dispense with the many semantic problems that surround the general concept of biological stress. One could safely assume that social stress is a definite set of behavioural and physiological responses specifically induced by the presence and/or particular actions (e.g. aggressive) of conspecifics. The traditional view, grounded on a great deal of research on domestic fowl, even specifies that social stress occurs during encounters between strangers or in crowded groups (Craig et al., 1969, begin their paper by stating that "strangeness and crowding are factors causing social stress"). Before this point is discussed, it is necessary to realize that a distinction between stressors and stress responses would be useful only if an adequate definition of stress was available, which is not the case (Freeman, 1987). As a general rule, stress is often given a circular definition in terms of either its causes (stressors) or its effects (physiological responses). For example, Craig (1981) states that: "Certain hormones show typical response patterns and cause symptomatic physiological changes in many situations that we consider as stressful. When those hormonal patterns or their physiological consequences are detected, it may reasonably be expected that one or more stressors are responsible".

As was mentioned earlier, the classical results from the research on domestic fowl, the farm species most extensively studied, have suggested that crowding and stangeness of the animals in presence were causes of social stress. This conclusion will now be examined, following Syme and Syme's (1974) general assertion that "social stress may be observed when the animal has to make abnormal or extreme physiological or behavioural adjustments in order to cope with its social environment".

## Crowding as a social stressor

Wood-Gush (1983) rightly noted that there is little evidence of social stress in farm livestock, so that he devoted only 3 pages to this topic in his book. He refers to some of the classical work on rodents, such as Christian's experiments on crowded or isolated mice, and Barnett's experiments on rats introduced as "interlopers" into pairs or groups of residents. Craig (1981) also referred to experiments with rodents showing that in males subjected to aggression from a conspecific, the effect of "psychological" stressors was at least as powerful as the effect of physical attacks in rising adrenorcortical response. As many authors, Craig implicitly refers to social stress as a variety of deleterious symptoms typically associated with crowding, and he mentions increase of adrenal weight as an indicator of such stress in some experiments carried out with chickens. Syme and Syme (1974) intimately relate social stress with crowding, to submit that "crowding always results in social stress. If the animals are not stressed, they do not perceive the particular social density as crowded".

Crowding cannot, by definition, be considered as a specific stressor. As such, it constitutes merely a biophysical factor susceptible to cause stress; it relates to density, i.e. to increase in group size, often together with a reduction in the floor area available to individuals. To count as a social stressor, such increase in the number of conspecifics per unit of space has to be perceived as critical or extreme, i.e. as overpopulation; also, this state of crowding should be followed by changes in the group social structure (e.g. dominance hierarchy). It is, therefore, rightly that crowding is sometimes classified as a "physical" stressor rather than as a "social" stressor (Freeman, 1987). As Siegel and Gross (1973) and Siegel (1976) have emphasized, crowding is not merely increased population density, a physical measure. Crowding is "a product of density, contact, communication and activity. It implies a pressure, a force, and a psychological reaction. Therefore, crowding may occur at widely different densities", and "results in social strife", or "cause social tension", or "increase social competition". So, in principle crowding could as well be investigated under the heading of social space (Zayan, 1985).

To conclude: density, as well as other (bio)physical variables, may cause social stress to the extent that they are associated with events perceived as causes of disturbance, as when an excessively increased group size coincides with the onset of aggressive interactions among the members of a formerly stable group. What is essential is that animals perceive increased density as crowding, and recognize its immediate effects as stressors arising from conspecifics. There is, thus, a cognitive or psychological process that transforms a (bio)physical situation into one of social stress. A priori, such cognitive mediation should be even more operative in the case of the next stressor to be discussed.

## Strangeness of conspecifics as a social stressor

It is well known that mixing unacquainted conspecifics usually induces reciprocal aggression, and that the onset of such fights increases adrenocortical responses. Farm animals are no exception in this respect (see e.g. Zayan, present volume, for the case of pigs). Perhaps the most classical illustration of social stress that one finds in the literature is provided by this experimental relationship: encounters among strangers (particularly showing biophysical and social symmetry) increase the activity of the pituitary-adrenocortical system via an increase of agonistic activities (aggressive and/or fear responses). It was suggested that the greatest stressor in moving cattle was agonistic encounters among unfamiliar individuals, because much fighting occurs during transportation (Price and Tennessen, 1981, quoted by Fraser and Rushen, 1987).

There are, however, several problems that make assertions such as these difficult to generalize. The first is that the specific effect of strangeness as a social stressor was never dissociated from its immediate behavioural effect, namely the induction of aggressive interactions. So, finding an increase in the levels of catecholamines and/or glucocorticoids cannot be attributed exclusively to the perception of conspecifics as strangers, independently of the reciprocal aggression that such detection induces. As it is often admitted, "among all forms of animals with a high degree of social organization, placing unacquainted individuals together is one of the most potent means of eliciting intense aggression" (Fraser and Rushen, 1987). Another major problem is that stangeness was hardly studied specifically, i.e. compared to a control condition of social familiarity, and tested in pairs or in groups of animals independently of the other factors which interacted with social strangeness in an uncontrolled manner. In chickens, stress among unfamiliar conspecifics was often studied with a view to cause social disruption, using procedures such as changing animals from their own stable group to another and rotating these strange chickens into various flocks. For example, plasma corticosterone levels were found to be much higher in the animals subjected to 2 weeks of systematic rotation than in the control individuals, maintained in their stable social hierarchy (Siegel and Gross, 1973). The levels of the adrenocortical responses so consistently varied in accordance with the amount of aggressive responses that the former could be chosen as single trait for a bidirectional selection, itself used in interaction with further high or low conditions of social stress (rotated or stable flocks, respectively), to brillantly demonstrate opposite resistance to bacterial infections and to viral diseases. The many results that have demonstrated an effect of increased aggression upon immunity to desease clearly show that social stress is not a chimerical concept, since it affects the genetic-hormonal makeup of (unfamiliar) individuals (Gross and Siegel, 1965 and 1973; Gross, 1984; Siegel and Latimer, 1975; Siegel, 1985; Blecha et al., 1985). Many of these results do not, however, demonstrate that social stress was induced by social strangeness because the experimental rotation of birds into groups of strangers creates all the other effects associated with the procedure of testing residents against intruders: more fear is imposed to the latter, because they are handled, carried, and introduced into an unfamiliar pen occupied by strange and aggressive residents, themselves familiar with each other (see Zayan, 1987a, for a methodological discussion on this artifact in poultry; see Zayan and Thinès, 1984, for a demonstration that social strangeness does induce physiological stress, whereas social familiarity reduces it).

Siegel and Siegel's (1961) Exp 3 is one of the rare specific tests carried out until now with domestic fowl. Males were introduced singly into pens containing 50 strange cocks each day for a period of 4 hours, during 22 days; the control birds were maintained in their own flock but were also handled and again introduced into their home pen with their 7 flockmates, in order to neutralize the environmental fear which was inevitable when the experimental birds were placed as intruders into the pens of strange, and most probably aggressive, residents. There still was an uncontrolled factor, namely that the experimental pens were already familiar to the flockmates, but unknown to the strange intruders. Besides, socially induced stress could not be specifically attributed to a difference between social strangeness and social familiarity, because group size probably also exerted different effects. As the authors noted, strongly different behavioural responses can be expected when an individual is being reunited with his 7 former groupmates, and when a newcomer is being immediately attacked by 50 strange residents. In any event, the left adrenals were found to be significantly heavier in the severely attacked strange intruders  than in the familiar members of  a stable groupe. Obviously,  a  lot of research remains  to be conducted on  the physiological stress induced  by the  properties of strange  conspecifics,  and  reduced by those of familiar ones.

The study of social discriminations should constitute a major topic in the future experimental research on social stress. As was already mentioned when the problem of crowding was discussed, it is difficult to identify effects of stress  without  ensuring that  the  stimuli  manipulated as  stressors  were actually perceived as such by the animals. A simple way to check that social strangeness induces stress is to contrast the target animal's behavioural and physiological  responses  towards  strangers  to  those  manifested  towards familiar conspecifics. Equivalently, to show that social strangeness acts as a specific stressor,  it  must be shown  that animals are  able to detect the strangeness  of conspecifics,  to which  they respond  by increased  adrenal activity and  by aggression,  whereas  they are at  the same time  capable to recognize other conspecifics as familiar  individuals,  to which they respond by decreased adrenal  activity and aggression. As  Freeman (1987)  observed, insufficient acknowledgement  is made of  perceptive matters when  effects of stressors are assessed. Recognition of familiar conspecifics as distinct from strangers is  one of  these perceptive components  of stress,  which Freeman considers as "psychological",  and could as well be  considered as cognitive components  of stress.  Freeman asks  himself whether  stressors" should  be identified as such only  if they have a psychological component.  If so then the potency of  any such stressor would  decline as the target  animal showed less developed powers  of memory,  imagination and foresight".  And,  as was suggested earlier,  the specific  effect of  social strangeness  as stressor should be tested as a perceptive event, i.e. by mere sensory exposure of the target animal to strange and to familiar conspecifics, independently of the direct behavioural contacts (usually aggressive interactions) that such strangeness tends to induce.

Finally, it has to be pointed out that the traditional assumption that social strangeness causes stress, whereas social familiarity would suppress it or decrease it, does not hold true. Suffice it to consider its logical equivalents: firstly, that lack of social stress implies social familiarity and, secondly, that occurrence of social stress implies social strangeness. Both are wrong: on the one hand, there are many non stressful situations that occur among strange conspecifics; on the other hand, many stressful situations occur among familiar conspecifics, even among those capable of individual recognition. Therefore, social strangeness is neither a necessary nor a sufficient condition for social stress to occur.

## Reduction of contact with conspecifics as a social stressor

In gregarious species such as domestic fowl, group-members and even unfamiliar conspecifics show a strong affiliative tendency. It seems, therefore, reasonable to assume that denial or interruption of social contact induces or increases stress.

The qualitative difference between presence and absence of social contact was investigated by Jones and Merry (1988), who took chicks reared in groups, and tested them individually or in pairs in an open field. They found latency to first steps to be shorter, and distress calls as well as defaecations to be significantly decreased, in the chicks tested as pairs. Besides, plasma corticosterone concentrations were found to be significantly increased in the chicks tested individually. These results suggest that the presence of a familiar conspecific reduced the novelty value of the open field as a situation inducing fear or emotionality in chicks, although an interpretation in terms of attempts to reinstate contact with former companions reared as group-members would require more experiments on the effects of separation upon distress. As a general rule, it is difficult to conclude that social contact reduces emotionality in chicks whereas isolated individuals would be under stress, as was shown e.g. by Savory and MacLeod's (1980) results contradicting earlier work on the effects of social facilitation.

Jones and Harvey (1987) investigated the quantitative differences that animals may perceive when the number of their cagemates is reduced, starting with groups of 8 chicks. They found that to progressive removal of companions corresponded significant increases in plasma corticosterone levels as well as in behavioural indices of fear, such as the number of distress calls and of defaecations. Again, disruption of the social environment was interpreted as eliciting fear or aversion in chicks. There is, however, a methodological problem when progressive reduction of group size is not followed by (or does not randomly alternate with) reestablishment of initial group size; there should also exist a control condition in which initial group size is kept constant whereas all the group-members are successively caught, taken out of the cage and reintroduced into it to be reunited with the other residents.

In a classical experiment, Siegel and Siegel (1961, Exp 4) tested adult males in 3 conditions: some were kept individually, in cages allowing the birds to see and hear some of their neighbours; others were continuously kept in groups of 5 birds; and others were alternately caged individually and placed in a 5-bird group for daily periods of 4 hrs, following the rotation procedure. Both the right and the left adrenals were found to be significantly heavier in the continuously grouped cocks than in those individually caged; the weight of the adrenals were intermediate in the birds grouped for only 4 hrs a day, their left adrenal being significantly heavier than those of permanent group-members. It is, however, difficult to conclude from this experiment that physiological stress tends to be increased by the social condition of permanent grouping, if only because all the birds had been individually caged during months previous to the experiments, and because strong differences existed between the cages of the separated birds and the pens where the permanent groups were formed. In addition, residents and intruders are differently treated in experiments using the rotation procedure.

To conclude, more experimental work is needed in order to confirm the hypothesis that the disruption of social relationships causes stress. Pairs and small groups of animals should be tested systematically in the future, because the members of large groups tend to form less stable relations as a result of decreased capacities to recognize various conspecifics.

## Aggression as a social stressor

Since old and anecdotal data by Guhl and Allee (1944), elevated rates of aggression have been associated and even equated with high levels of social stress. As was already mentioned, such association was taken for granted under conditions which tend to promote social tension, as when many conspecifics are grouped for the very first time or when strangers are being added to stable groups (Craig, 1981). Other conditions have been used to induce aggression, implicitly with an aim to induce social stress. A typical example is  competitive situations,   as when food  is presented  in one-hole troughs following a critical period of deprivation. Early ethologists willing to find  out peck-orders in  groups of domestic  fowl often resorted  to such competitive  tests whenever  they  failed  to observe  spontaneous  agonistic interactions among the members of stable flocks.  It is very likely that such experimentally induced aggression corresponded  to situations inducing social stress.  However,  it would be erroneous to believe,  as is traditionally the case,  that competitive  situations necessarily induce aggression,  and that they also  necessarily induce  social stress.  Social stress  was too  often confused with  competition and conflict,  and  the two latter were  too often confused  with the  onset of  aggression.  Clearly,  aggression  is not  the privileged means for animals to solve a  conflict when faced to a competitive situation.  In  domestic fowl,  familiar members  of a stable  peck-order may share restricted  resources and  cope with  many a  competitive situation  by cooperative  behaviour. Since  aggressive  responses  may be  manifested  in contexts  other  than  competitive,  the  two  notions  of  aggression  and competition should be definitely dissociated.

Competition does, however, induce conflict which, in turn,  may or may not be  solved by  aggression.  It may be  admitted  that  many non  aggressive behavioural solutions to psychological conflict  do not elicit social stress. Consequently,  neither competition  nor  conflict  necessarily cause  social stress,  and therefore should  not be associated with the latter  as they too often are  in the literature,  because the  cases where conflict  results in aggression  are overemphasized.  And,  as  a general  rule,  it  is fair  to postulate that aggression  induces social stress: fighting  is undoubtedly a stressful  experience  (Huntingford and  Turner,  1987),  and agonistic interactions undoubtedly elicit fear in the target animal subjected to repeated attacks. In contrast, it is not true that animals experience social stress exclusively in aggressive contexts. Besides, it would be wrong to infer that occurrence of social stress necessarily implies that animals engage in overt aggression. Equivalently, lack of overt aggression does not imply that animals do not currently undergo social stress. Non aggressive animals may be in a state of stress that they manifest by other conflict behaviours.

Because social stress does not necessarily imply competition, nor conflict, nor even aggression, it should be investigated in contexts other than those promoting competition, conflict, or aggression. The concept of psychological or social conflict seems the most general to which social stress could be attached. Indeed, whereas it is true that competition causes conflict, not all conflict results from competition; and, whereas it is true that aggression always corresponds to some conflict, not all conflict results in aggression.

To conclude: aggression is not, by itself, a relevant indicator of social stress. It is, instead, a reliable indicator of the animals' relative state of aggressiveness; in the case of an animal unilaterally subjected to aggression, flight responses are a reliable indicator of the animal's psychological state of (social) fear and, perhaps, of its physiological state of (social) stress. In all cases, increased frequency and/or intensity of agonistic interactions, and even induction of reciprocal aggression, are never direct indicators of social stress. These behavioural events have to be related to concomitant increases in the levels of measures indicative of physiological stress, particularly to elevations of catecholamines and/or corticosteroid concentrations. In contrast, increase in the frequency and/or intensity of aggressive interactions will more specifically be related to concomitant increases in the levels of testosterone and of other physiological indicators of aggressiveness and/or social fear.

## Aggressive status as a social stressor

The abusive association made in the literature between social stress and aggression has led to dubious suggestions, such as that stress may be greater in the more aggressive hens and in the dominant strains of birds, whereas it would be less pronounced in the less aggressive hens and in the more submissive strains. What may be true for increased aggression may not apply to higher status in the dominance hierarchy even if, as noted by Wood-Gush (1971), it may be just as stressful to maintain a high position as to be kept in a low social status. However, the more stressed individuals may not be the more aggressive ones. Siegel and Siegel (1961) did not find that the weights of the adrenals were clearly correlated with winning or losing aggressive pair encounters with a stranger, nor did the authors find any significant correlation between adrenal changes and social rank in members of small flocks with a more or less stable peck-order. Marsteller et al. (1980) have also shown that during the formation of peck-orders physiological stress, indicated by plasma corticosterone concentrations, was not significantly correlated with the frequency of encounters lost or won. Wood-Gush (1971) was right in suggesting that a straightforward correlation should not be expected between the state of the adrenals and the peck-order position of fowls. The main reason for this is semantic: social dominance is not the same as aggressive behaviour; aggression is not the same as aggressiveness; the latter is not the same as another internal state, social stress. Thus, animals subjected to social stress may well be aggressive but not manifest overt aggression. For example, subordinate hens, or birds with intermediate social rank may so be inhibited by the potential aggression of dominants; Ylander and Craig (1980) have shown such inhibition of agonistic interactions among domestic hens by the near presence of a dominant and occasionally threatening flockmate. Cognitive processes such as visual attention and social recognition may control, i.e. facilitate or inhibit, the initiation of overt aggression.

## Hormonal indicators

The problem discussed here is not whether hormonal responses are more or less reliable indicators of stress than are other physiological effects, e.g. increase in the levels of circulating eosinophil leukocytes (Heller et al., 1988; see also Gross and Siegel, 1983, for a similar suggestion that a marked and stable increase in number of heterophil leukocytes after social stress may provide a more consistent assessment of stress in chickens than corticosteroid elevation). Rather, the issue raised will concern the need to distinguish hormonal responses other than those recorded after stressful experiences such as fighting or defeat following fights. As will be seen, hormonal indicators of social stress can hardly be dissociated from those of agonistic events in a great deal of the recent literature, and it was suggested earlier that social stressors should not be restricted to aggressive inputs. Besides, it will be apparent that hormonal responses are equivocal indicators, for they often reflect at the same time an increase in aggression and the outcomes of aggressive encounters.

It is hard to deny that aggressiveness is under the control of androgens in Vertebrates, although the effect of testosterone is complicated by the social context where aggression occurs, and by the fighting experience itself (see Huntingford and Turner, 1987, for an excellent review of hormonal correlates of aggression and social stress, and from which many examples were borrowed). In blackbirds, for example, testosterone levels are very high in the most aggressive of the fighting birds, and very low in the birds showing more fearful responses (Harding and Follett, 1979; Harding, 1983); intense variations of hormonal levels are particularly recorded during fights for the possession of a territory. In simulated territorial intrusions, male sparrows trying to acquire a territory have higher testosterone levels than males having already a territory, intrusion being an event that increases testosterone. And, castrated sparrows implanted with testosterone are not more aggressive as they are observed in their stable groups, but a transient increase of aggressiveness is manifested towards unfamiliar birds (Wingfield and Ramenofsky, 1985). These data simply confirm what the behavioural data have shown, namely that familiar birds are aggressive towards strangers, and that residents are aggressive towards intruders.

Although testosterone levels fairly correlate with readiness to initiate a fight, in many Vertebrates (e.g. rats, mice or Rhesus monkeys), androgen levels are raised at the same time in aggressive and in dominant individuals, and lowered at the same time in their less aggressive and subordinate counterparts. Initially, short-term increases in testosterone occur at the start of a fight, and contribute to produce escalated fights, especially in opponents whose initial level of testosterone was equivalent; the enhanced production of testosterone facilitates and maintains fighting, thus probably

short-terms stress.    After the   fights,   the hormonal  state differs   in the

dominant and in defeated animal because   testosterone levels remain higher in

the former and critically fall in the latter.  As a general rule,   changes in

agonistic status   are reflected  by changes  in androgen  levels,   as   can be

checked   when dominants  are experimentally  made  submissive or   conversely.

Interestingly,  dominant  and subordinate  male Baboons  may show  equivalent

testosterone levels in   normal conditions,   but androgen levels  will rise in

the dominants and fall in the subordinates if animals are subjected to stress

(Sapolsky, 1982).   In male Japanese quail fighting for the first time, plasma

corticosterone levels   correlate with aggression  before and after   the first

fight;  but,  as the dominance-subordination relations are established during

subsequent encounters,   the testosterone levels become lower in the dominants

than in the subordinates (Ramenofsky, 1984; Wingfield and Ramenofsky, 1985).

   Results on testosterone are relevant to  the problem of social stress only

because high androgen levels seem to clearly contribute to enhance aggression

(as  well as  aggressive dominance),   and because  reciprocal aggression  is

undoubtedly  a stressful  experience.  However,   increased  aggression  (and

enhanced  potential to  win fights)  are actually  behavioural (and  social)

indicators of  higher aggressiveness,   not necessarily  of increased  social

stress.  To the contrary,  animals showing  less or no aggression and animals

with a submissive  agonistic status are those for which  it should reasonably

be assumed that they undergo a higher social stress.  Here, it must be turned

to data on  adrenal hormones in order  to check how agonistic  encounters and

their  outcomes (victory   or  defeat)  relate  to  physiological  stress.

Subordinate and less  aggressive animals showing lower  androgen levels after

the stress of  fights,  should in principle show  higher catecholamine and/or

glucocorticoid levels in comparison to their dominant counterparts.

First, it is clearly the case that fighting causes stress. In rodents, both the levels of catecholamines and the levels of glucocorticoids are increased during fights; after the encounters, however, subordinates have higher adrenaline levels than dominants (whereas these have higher noradrenaline levels and higher noradrenaline:adrenaline ratios), and the increase of corticosterone is stronger and longer lasting in the defeated animals (Brain, 1980; Schuurman, 1980).

So, assessing the relation between social stress and catecholamines seems to require that changes in adrenaline and in noradrenaline be distinguished. Such distinction is not always made, as when it is found that the brains of mice from spontaneously aggressive strains contain higher catecholamine levels than do those of less aggressive animals (Serri and Ely, 1984). In rodents, the following general mechanisms can be described to account for hormonal control of agonistic stressful experience (Huntingford and Turner, 1987): – Glucocorticoids indirectly increase aggression, by negative feedback inhibiting ACTH production; initially ACTH facilitates aggression but, in the long term, it directly inhibits it. – Glucocorticoids directly facilitate subordination and submissive responses; ACTH also (indirectly) enhances submission, by increasing glucocorticoid production (injecting ACTH or cortocosteroids to subordinates increases and accelerates their submissiveness ;Leshner, 1983).

The picture is also rather clear with other Vertebrates. Thus in male fish figting in pairwise encounters, both opponents show a rapid increase in their plasma corticosteroid levels, but this effect is weaker and shorter in the winner than in the loser, so that the dominant eventually shows lower levels of corticosterone (whereas the subordinate shows lower testosterone levels;

Hannes et al., 1984). In voles, subordinate males most subjected to attacks suffer from anatomical and physiological impairments as a result of increased adrenal activity during stressful encounters (Rasa and Vandenhoovel, 1984). It was often found that a deficit in immunological response was increased as a result of defeat following fights. As a general rule, it can be concluded that animals exposed to severe or repeated submission undergo social stress.

The relationship between adrenal hormones, indicative of physiological stress, and agonistic experience, traditionally considered as a privileged source of social stress, is far from being straightforward. Fighting modifies the production of pituitary-adrenal hormones, these influence the intensity and outcomes of fights, and in turn the outcomes affect the levels of catecholamine and adrenocortical responses. So, "stress hormones" are certainly affected by, and they affect, aggression-dependent social stress. But they also are affected by social experience associated with winning or losing fights, as well as by many other factors such as the relative stability of the group in which fights occur. In monkeys, high glucocorticoid concentrations are found in the animals becoming progressively dominant as agonistic encounters occur in the course of hierarchy formation; once the hierarchy has been established, the dominants show lower glucocorticoid levels. Development also plays a role in calibrating the levels of adrenocortical responses to be later associated with high agonistic status: subadult Rhesus monkeys have a greater chance to win fights if their plasma glucocorticoid concentrations are low than if they are elevated (Golub et al., 1979).

To conclude this section, it is obvious that hormones differentially control two types of social stress dependent upon aggressive experience:

fighting, and social status resulting from fights. What remains to be made are many etho-endocrinological experiments in which could be investigated the hormonal correlates of social stress induced in contexts other than those of agonistic encounters.

## An integrative approach

The main reason why the concept of social stress remains in the twilight is that it implicitly belongs to 3 levels of reality (Figure 1).

First, it is obvious that animals subjected to social stress are exposed to certain conspecifics, even if they are not always members of a stable group or society. So in one way or another, they take part in a social structure and belong to some social system. At this sociological level of analysis, the degree of stress depends on some of the properties exclusively possessed by the system composed of a set of conspecifics, their structure or organization (i.e. the set of their relations), and their immediate social and physical environment. Thus, social stress will be increased by instability, poor cohesion and loose integration, counting as some of the emergent properties of a set of interacting conspecifics. And, social stress will be explained by some emergent properties of the social structure, e.g. by strong or sudden competition, by a tendency towards segregative differentiation, or by abrupt changes in statuses or roles leading to restructuring through increased social mobility. In Primates, the stress of individuals depends not just upon the quality of the interactions among the group-members but also on the cultural or the economical structure of the society (e.g. participative or segregative; Hinde, 1982).

FIGURE 1

## LEVELS OF ANALYSIS OF SOCIAL STRESS

SOCIAL SYSTEMS                    SOCIOLOGICAL

Emergent properties :
stability, cohesion, integration

Explanatory processes :
differentiation — participation
competition — cooperation
social mobility — social inertia

SOCIAL SUBSYSTEMS               PSYCHOLOGICAL

Explanatory processes
(oocial mechanisms) :

* Cognitive connections
  social recognition (familiar - strange)
  individual recognition

* Emotional couplings
  social fear, aggressiveness

BEHAVIOURAL

Descriptive-predictive animal interactions
(social indicators)

INDIVIDUAL SUBSYSTEMS      Organic responses to social stressors :

Behavioural, Neural (neuropsychological,
neuroethological), Physiological (hormones,
metabolism, immunity), Genetic, etc.

The second level of analysis refers to the subsets of conspecifics composing a group or society: tetrads, triads, but in any case at least pairs and not individuals. Indeed, the subsystems of a social system have to possess social properties not possessed by single organisms. These emergent properties and processes require to be analyzed at the interindividual level of social relations and connections among the group's components. Among the possible connections, one thinks immediately of behavioural interactions, such as those described in aggressive encounters; in turn, behavioural interactions may serve as indicators of social relations, as when stable and unilateral agonistic encounters permit to infer that the animal showing consistent aggression is dominant over the animal responding submissively by repeated flights. But it is generally overlooked that behavioural interactions are controlled, i.e. either facilitated or inhibited, by other interindividual processes not directly observable. These are the set of elementary cognitive couplings and their emotional correlates which affect each of the conspecific's state. For example, social stress will be enhanced if opponents detect each other as strangers; it will be reduced if conspecifcs recognize each other as familiar group-members or as particular individuals, and if they recognize each other as conspecifics associated with a past and persistent dominance or subordination experience. Enhanced social stress will correspond to increased aggressiveness and/or social fear. It must be emphasized that the cognitive and emotional couplings form a set of intervening variables (more precisely, of hypothetical constructs referring to definite neurophysiological processes) capable to explain the occurrence of behaviours indicative of social stress. Thus, social recognition will inhibit aggression towards familiar conspecifics, and elicit aggression towards strangers. Similarly, social fear towards a stranger perceived as too much advantaged by body weight will override aggresssiveness, as will the latter be inhibited in subordinates recognizing their former dominant. In other words, behaviour possibly indicative of social stress can be explained by psychological processes. These are social mechanisms in their own right, for they occur "in the mind" (and in the brain) of a set of socially connected individuals. The couplings or connections among animals need not always be observable behavioural interactions (see Dawkins, 1985 and Zayan, 1987b for such a claim). And, as will now be shown, interactions and connections at the interindividual (social) level may be explained by organic processes at the level of individuals.

Individuals lack the emergent properties of social systems (groups or societies) and of social subsystems (at least dyads of conspecifics, together with their interindividual connections, i.e. behavioural interactions as well as cognitive/emotional couplings). For this reason, processes occurring in single organisms fail to count as relevant mechanisms of social behaviour and cognition. Thus, a group's social instability, associated with increased aggression of its members, cannot be directly explained by the neuroendocrine activity and by other internal processes of each group-member. But an indirect explanation will be achieved, in the case of social stress, provided that: - specific social stressors have been selected and identified, by means of systematic experiments controlling the properties of conspecifics inducing stress; - specific stress responses to experimentally controlled social stressors have been consistently recorded and identified. In that case, individuals and their organic states will count as relevant subsystems of the interindividual reality social stress constitutes. Hopefully, the set of internal processes of the animal(s) acting as social stressor(s) will, at least partly, differ from the set of organic responses recorded in the target animal(s) subjected to social stress. The preceding section on hormonal responses indicates that in the context of agonistic stress, the neuroendocrine profile of aggressive dominants is quite distinct from that of their aggressed subordinates. Future research will have to seek for other differences between the neural, physiological, immunological or genetic states of the animals causing stress, and the corresponding states of their conspecifics coping with it. The distinct behavioural patterns of the stressing and of the stressed animals can also be separately analyzed as responses of organisms at the individual level. The same as with the cognitive (e.g. recognition of a former dominant) and with the emotional (e.g. fear towards an aggressive stranger) internal processes of each individual, the peripheral behaviours of each animal can be analyzed in terms of internal organic states. Because stress occurring in agonistic contexts was previously discussed, the case of dominance-subordination relationships will now serve to illustrate the integrative view being proposed here as a strategy for future research (see Figure 2). Dominants may be subjected to constant social stress in defending their status. Although an aggresive dominant may also subject a subordinate to constant stress, the two animals will still maintain a bond that will reflect the social structure to which they belong as dyads. Thus, the degree of stability of their dominance relation will reflect the degree of linearity of the group's dominance hierarchy.

FIGURE 2

SOCIOLOGICAL LEVEL
( stable social relationships, personal bonds )

Dominant ($\alpha$) status          Subordinate ($\omega$) status

INTERINDIVIDUAL LEVEL
( social relations and connections )

Agonistic $\alpha$ status          Agonistic $\omega$ status

Behavioural
interactions

Agonistic $\alpha$ states          Agonistic $\omega$ states
( Aggression )          ( Flight )

Cognitive
couplings

Agonistic $\alpha$ experience          Agonistic $\omega$ experience

recognition:          of a former $\alpha$ or $\omega$ conspecific
attribution:          of an $\alpha$ or $\omega$ agonistic state
          of an $\alpha$ or $\omega$ potential status

learning:          set of $\alpha$ behaviours          set of $\omega$ behaviours
preference:          for an $\omega$ cooperator          for an $\alpha$ protector

INTRAINDIVIDUAL LEVEL
( internal organic states )

Hormonal          Aggressiveness          Social fear & stress

Neural          Awareness of aggressive state          Awareness of fear state

          Propension to fight          Propension to flight
Genetic          Predisposition to dominate          Predisposition to submit
          Bodily resistance          Susceptibility to injuries

At the sociological level, dominants and subordinates are connected by a relationship, i.e. by unilateral agonistic interactions possessing the property of stability, complementarity, and familiarity among the related animals of dominant and subordinate status (Hinde, 1982). At the interindividual level, relations and connections are established between socially differentiated individuals. To the agonistic status of dominant and to the agonistic status of subordinate correspond, respectively: - the agonistic state of aggression and the agonistic state of flight or avoidance, at the descriptive level of behaviour interactions; - an agonistic experience of dominance and an agonistic experience of submission, as well as recognition between former dominants and subordinates, at the level of (unobservable) cognitive couplings. Finally, at the individual level, i.e. at the level of intra-individual organic processes, to the behavioural states of aggression and of flight correspond, respectively: - hormonal states of aggressiveness and of social fear (or of social stress); - neural activities such as awareness of being in an aggressive state or in a state of fear; - genetic tendencies, such as propension to fight or to flight, predisposition to dominate or to submit, and increased bodily resistance or increased susceptibility to injuries and diseases.

It is presently submitted that only a multilevel approach to social stress will adequately grasp the emergent properties of this complex process, and correctly attempt to explain them by acknowledging their ethological (behavioural) and psychological (cognitive) mechanisms. Skipping these intermediate levels, by directly collecting hormonal and other internal measures at the level of single organisms, is reductionism. It may disclose mechanisms of physiological stress, but these will be irrelevant to explain   social stress.

## Social stress in small groups of laying hens

In accordance  with some of  the traditional  assumptions to which  it was
earlier referred  in this paper,   it can be  admitted that social  stress is
enhanced,  particularly  in gregarious species  such as domestic  fowl,  when
animals cannot form a stable group and develop activities tending to maximize
the group's  cohesion.  In  contrast,  social  stress would  be decreased  in
situations where animals can manifest  affiliative behaviour that brings  them
and keeps them together.  Usually, socially attracted conspecifics eventually
develop personal bonds;   what maintains stable relationships  among familiar
individuals is  cooperative behaviour,   even in  conflict situations.   As a
general rule, permanent bodily contact,  inhibition of aggression and lack of
avoidance behaviour suggest  that social stress is reduced  among the members
of a group.  In principle,   highly individualized relationships,  associated
both with social stability and with social cooperation,  should correspond to
a decrease  in adrenocortical  responses indicative of  social stress.   In a
species such as domestic fowl,  visual attention certainly operates to ensure
a perceptive control of the activities  of familiar conspecifics.  This,  and
other  elementary  cognitive  processes,   contribute  to  avoid  agonistic
encounters and  to promote behaviour  beneficial to  others.  So,  it  may be
submitted that social  stress would occur in situations  where animals cannot
develop personal bonds and achieve cooperation.  Social stress would,  by the
same token,  coindice with a  breakdown of the cognitive/emotional mechanisms
by which  groupmates achieve coordinated  activities that may  increase their
welfare, even under restricted environmental conditions. In the experiment to

be now reported, the animals were subjected to a restriction of the space available in their cages. The smallest possible groups of laying hens were formed, namely triads, to which were compared the simplest (i.e. also the most basic) social systems, namely pairs of animals. Previous research on the social space of laying hens housed in battery-like experimental cages revealed that aggression was nearly totally absent and interindividual distances were extremely short, among members of pairs observed in conditions ranging from severe confinement to very large available space per hen. The pair-members tended to manifest affiliative behaviour resulting in frequent bodily contacts. These results were interpreted in terms of the pair condition tending to maximize social stability and social cohesion among cagemates, mainly as a result of their highly coordinated behaviour. Accordingly, the hypothesis was made that groups of hens would behave as less integrated social systems because, given the same floor area per animal as were the pairs, the members of groups would compete more for restricted space (Zayan et al., 1983). This hypothesis was later confirmed by a long-term experiment comparing pairs with randomly selected dyads from groups of 4 hens. In the latter, the interindividual distances were significantly larger, and the frequency of agonistic interactions was significantly higher than in the former (Zayan and Doyen, 1985). Because aggressive hierarchies were sometimes formed among the groups of hens, it was supposed that the possible dyadic stable relations formed within these tetrads were complicated by individuals of intermediate status maintaining social tension. In the pairs, no third party could possible interfere with the highly sociable partners sharing the cage. This suggestion was tested by using triads and was carried on further by recording not only the behaviour and physical distances among individuals, but also the adrenocortical responses indicative of higher social stress.

Laying hens of 2 commercial strains (W: White Leghorn, R: Rhode Island Red hybrids) were housed for a period of 10 months in experimental battery-like cages whose floors could be varied in order to provide the birds with constant area in groups of different sizes. It was decided to allow 600 $cm^2$/bird, because such floor area approximates to those recently mentioned as minimum space required for hens in current European farms. Birds had previously been reared in battery cages, and beak-trimmed at the age of 10 days. Observations were made using closed-circuit video cameras placed above the cages. 12 cages were observed in each condition during 5 periods of 20 minutes per cage and per month.

Agonistic interactions were recorded at very low frequencies; they were in most cages observed for the first time during the 5th month. Aggression was nearly never recorded among the R hens; pecks, manifested alone or in association with threats, were significantly more frequent among the members of triads than among those of pairs in the W hens (Table 1). If all types of agonistic acts are considered (Table 2), these similarly increased in the pairs and in the triads of W hens, but occurred more frequently among the members of triads than among those of pairs in the R hens. Interestingly, among these hens of the R strain the pair-members addressed a significantly higher number of pecks to the hens of their adjacent cages than did the members of triads (U=36, p<0.025, Mann-Whitney test; p=0.05, Fisher test); such result was not found for the W hens. The members of the R strain (but not those of the W strain) also executed more allo-preening in pairs than in triads (U=42, p=0.05; p=0.005, Fisher test).

These data are consistent with those of all agonistic acts. In the hens of the R strain, individuals devote less attention to peck, threat or push away their only partner than another group-member, but they concentrate more on their partner than on a group-member to engage in a behaviour of mutual benefit which also tends to strengthen social bonds. Conversely, the members of pairs redirect their aggression towards their neighbours, usually jumping in order to deliver their pecks over their metal partitions of the cage; in contrast, the members of the triads devote more attention to deliver aggressive acts to their cagemates and are less interested in pecking at the members of their adjacent cages.

The fact that agonistic interactions were more frequently observed among the members of triads should indicate that interindividual distances were actually smaller among the members of pairs, since aggressive pecks and threats normally cause a cagemate to flee or move away. Similarly, more frequent allo-preening among pair-members should correspond with more frequent contacts. These indications were statistically confirmed, both for the case of contacts (W hens: $p<0.005$, R hens: $p=0.01$) and for the case of mean distances recorded between cagemates (W hens: $p<0.001$, R hens: $p<0.002$). The physical measures of interindividual distances were assessed following a method described elsewhere (Zayan and Doyen, 1985). The values mentioned for triads in Table 3 refer to distances recorded among selected dyads within the groups. The first values report the mean distances recorded between the same two selected birds, and they include successive interposition of the other cagemate; the second and third values, indicated between parentheses, correspond to the distances recorded between one selected bird and, respectively, each of the other two nearest and each of the other two farthest group-members.

Mortality percentages and defeathering scores, expressed as percentage of total missing plumage assessed by estimated defeathered areas of 10 body tracts, were compared in 48 pairs and in 48 triads of each strain, following the method described by Herremans et al. (see their paper in the present volume). As can be seen on Table 4, mortality rates were low and did not differ significantly in the pairs and in the triads, whereas defeathering was about twice more pronounced among the members of triads as among the members of pairs. This difference, slightly significant (p=0.048) 1 month after the end of the observation period, is very clear after the birds were left for 5 additional months in their cages (Table 4): in the birds of the two strains, overall mortality rates and defeathering scores were significantly higher among the members of triads (p<0.01). The latter result was mainly due to a severe state of defeathering observed among the members of the triads of the R strain, particularly at parts of the body corresponding to the abdominal-anal, caudal, and dorsopelvic tracts. These areas are typically defeathered by pecking that tends to precede cannibalism, an indication confirmed by the fact that feather pecking started to be frequently observed in the R triads during the 10th month, and that half of the dead birds in these R triads were actually killed by continuous chasing. It was only in the W and in the R triads that screams were emitted by pecked birds continously forced to flee.

Finally, no significant differences between pairs and triads were found concerning egg production until the 11th month. However, the members of the pairs produced more eggs than those of the triads after a laying period of 16 months; this difference (+ 4,1%, p=0.019, U-test) was most significant if egg production per initial hen, rather than per hen present, is considered (+ 5,9%, p=0.009 and p=0.006 for comparisons on the number of cages and on the number of hens, respectively).

From these experiments, conducted with normally beak-trimmed hens, it can be concluded that recommendations about minimum floor space for laying hens in battery cages should not be attempted independently of group-size. In this respect, the results confirm our previous recommendations after experiments which compared pairs of hens with groups of 4 hens provided with the same floor area (545cm$^2$, or 850 cm$^2$ per bird), namely that it would be preferable to house pairs rather than groups of hens in battery cages providing a floor space close to the restricted areas of the current intensive cages.

A final result suggests that welfare may be increased, and social stress be reduced, in hens housed in pairs in battery cages. When the hens of the two strains were taken out of their cages after 16 months of residence in their cages, plasma corticosterone concentrations, which are considered to be reliable indicators of physiological stress, were found to be very significantly higher among the hens kept as pairs than among those kept as triads. This result was found for the 2 strains(see Table 5). So, separation from just one cagemate seems to be more stressful than leaving a cage with two other familiar conspecifics. This result suggests that pair-members develop more bonding relations with each other than do the members of triads. Social disruption seems, therefore, to be more tolerated by the members of triads. As a matter of fact, it is only in the cages containing triads that severe aggressive behaviour, causing flights and shrieks, was recorded from the 13th month onwards. No chasing behaviour, nor strong avoidances, were ever observed among the members of pairs even after 16 months of residence in the battery cages.

TABLE 1. Median values of all agonistic pecks (+ threats) recorded in each cage (600cm$^2$/bird) among dyads of hens observed during 10 months (5 observation periods of 20 min. per cage and per month).

|  | R Hens | | W Hens | |
| --- | --- | --- | --- | --- |
| Members of: | Pairs | Triads | Pairs | Triads |
|  | – | – | – | – |
|  | – | – | – | 1 (+1) |
|  | – | – | – | 2 |
|  | – | – | – | 3 |
|  | – | – | – | 3 |
|  | – | – | – | 3 |
|  | – | – | – | 3 |
|  | – | – | 1 | 3 (+2) |
|  | – | – | 1 | 7 (+1) |
|  | – | – | 1 | 9 (+1) |
|  | – | – | 2 | 10 |
|  | – | 1 | 30 | 13 |
| Fisher test | p>0.05 | | p=0.025 | |
| U    test pecks | p>0.05 | | U=22,5 p<0.005 | |
| pecks + threats | p>0.05 | | U=20,5 p<0.001 | |

TABLE 2. Median values of all agonistic acts recorded in each cage (600 cm²/bird) among dyads of hens observed during 10 months (5 observation periods of 20 min per cage and per month). Pecks, threats, and acts forcing a cagemate to move away (scratch, leg hit).

| Members of: | R Hens | | W Hens | |
| --- | --- | --- | --- | --- |
| | Pairs | Triads | Pairs | Triads |
| | – | – | – | 2 |
| | – | – | – | 2 |
| | – | – | – | 3 |
| | – | – | 2 | 3 |
| | – | 1 | 2 | 4 |
| | – | 1 | 4 | 6 |
| | – | 1 | 4 | 8 |
| | – | 3 | 5 | 11 |
| | – | 4 | 6 | 11 |
| | 1 | 4 | 7 | 14 |
| | 1 | 8 | 14 | 14 |
| | 1 | 11 | 30 | 24 |
| Fisher test | p=0.05 | | p>0.05 | |
| U test | U=34, p<0.025 | | p>0.05 | |

TABLE 3. Mean interindividual distances and mean number of contacts recorded in cages of hens kept in pairs or in triads (5 observation periods of 20 min per month and per cage).
Hens of 2 strains (W= White Leghorn; R= Rhode Island Red) kept in battery cages with 600 cm² floor area per bird.
N= 12 cages in each condition.

| | Contacts | | Interindividual distances | |
| --- | --- | --- | --- | --- |
| | Pairs | Triads | Pairs | Triads |
| W Hens Means | 307 | 169 | 0,4 | 5,5 (2,4-2,9) |
| | 27 | 20 | 0,1 | 1,0 |
| R Hens Means | 267 | 204 | 0,1 | 4,1 (1,4-2,0) |
| | 19 | 35 | 0,08 | 1,7 |

TABLE 4. Mortality % and mean defeathering scores (% of total body plumage) in laying hens of 2 strains (W: White Leghorn; R: Rhode Island Red) kept in battery cages (n=2 or n=3) for a period of 11 months (above) and of 16 months (below). N=48 cages per condition.

| Strain: | W Hens | | R Hens | |
|---|---|---|---|---|
| | Pairs | Triads | Pairs | Triads |
| Area/bird: | $600cm^2$ | $600cm^2$ | $600cm^2$ | $600cm^2$ |
| Mortality % | 0 | 3,5 | 0 | 0 |
| Defeathering | 5,8 | 11,3 | 7,3 | 13,1 |
| Area/bird: | $600cm^2$ | $600cm^2$ | $600cm^2$ | $600cm^2$ |
| Mortality % | 2,1 | 6,9 | 3,3 | 9 |
| Defeathering % total body | 7,8 | 16,8 | 9,5 | 22,7 |
| % A+C+D areas | 10,9 | 16,7 | 12,6 | 31,6 |

A+C+D areas: Abdominal-anal, caudal, dorsopelvic tracts.

TABLE 5. Median values of plasma corticosterone levels (ng/ml) of laying hens of 2 strains (W and R). Blood samples taken after 62 weeks of residence in battery cages, either in pairs or in triads. W: White Leghorn, R: Rhode Island Red. Comparisons made using Mann-Whitney U-tests.

|  | Hens kept in Triads | Hens kept in Pairs |
|---|---|---|
| W Hens |  |  |
| N = | 40 | 32 |
| Medians | 2,4 | 4,9 |
| Comparison | z = 4,04 | p <0.0001 |
|  |  |  |
| R Hens |  |  |
| N = | 36 | 32 |
| Medians | 2,5 | 4,3 |
| Comparison | z = 2,60 | p = 0.005 |

REFERENCES

Blecha, F., Pollmann, D.S. and Nichols, D.A. 1985. Immunologic reactions of pigs regrouped at or near weaning. Am. J. Vet. Res., 46, 1934-1937.

Brain, P.F. 1980. Adaptive aspects of humoral correlates of attack and defeat in laboratory mice: a study in ethobiology. Rec. Progr. Br. Res., 53, 391-413.

Craig, J.V. 1981. Domestic Animal Behaviour. Prentice Hall.

Craig, J.V., Biswas, D.K. and Guhl, A.M. 1969. Agonistic behaviour influenced by strangeness, crowding and heredity in female domestic fowl (Gallus gallus). Anim. Behav., 17, 498-506.

Dawkins, M.S. 1985. Social space: the need for a new look at animal communication. In "Social Space for Domestic Animals", R. Zayan (ed), Martinus Nijhoff Publishers for the C.E.C., pp. 15-22.

Fraser, D. and Rushen, J. 1987. Aggressive behaviour. In "Farm Animal Behaviour", E.O. Price (ed), Veterinary Clinics of North America. vol 3, n°2, pp. 285-305.

Freeman, B.M. 1987. The stress syndrome. World Poultry Sci. J., 43, 15-19.

Golub, M.S., Sassenrath, E.N. and Goo, G.P. 1979. Plasma cortisol levels and dominance in peer groups of Rhesus monkeys weanlings. Horm. Behav., 12, 50-59.

Gross, W.B. and Siegel, H.S. 1965. The effect of social stress on resistance to infection with E. coli or M. gallisepticum. Poultry Sci., 44, 998-1001.

Gross, W.B. and Siegel, P.B. 1973. Effect of social stress and steroids on antibody production. Avian Dis., 17, 807-815.

Gross, W.B. and Siegel, H.S. 1983. Evaluation of the heterophil/lymphocyte ratio as a measure of stress in chickens. Avian Dis., 27, 972-979.

Gross, W.B. 1984. Effect of a range of social stress severity on E. coli challenge infection. Am. J. Vet. Res., 45, 2074-2076.

Guhl, A.M. and Allee, W.C. 1944. Some measurable effects of social organization in hens. Physiol. Zool., 17, 320-347.

Hannes, R.P., Franck, D. and Liemann, F. 1984. Effects of rank order fights on whole-body and blood concentrations of androgens and corticosteroids in the male swordtail (Xiphophorus helleri). Zeit. Tierpsychol., 65, 53-64.

Harding, C.F. 1983. Hormonal influences on avian aggressive behaviour. In "Hormones and Aggressive Behaviour", B.B. Svare (ed), Plenum Press, pp. 435-467.

Harding,  C.F.  and  Follett,  B.K.  1979.  Hormone  changes  triggerred  by aggression in a natural population of blackbirds. Science, 203, 918-920.

Heller, K.E., Houbak, B. and Jeppesen, L.L. 1988. Stress during mother-infant separation in ranch mink. Behav. Processes, 17, 217-227.

Hinde, R.A. 1982. Ethology. Oxford University Press.

Huntingford, F.A. and Turner, A.K. 1987. Animal Conflict. Chapman and Hall.

Jones, R.B. and Harvey, S. 1987.  Behavioural and adrenocortical responses of domestic chicks to systematic reductions in  group size and to sequential disturbance of companions  by the experimenter.  Behav.   Processes,  14, 291-303.

Jones, R.B. and Merry, B.J.  1988.  Individual or paired exposure of domestic chicks  to  an  open  field:  some  behavioural  and  adrenocortical consequences. Behav. Processes, 16, 75-86.

Leshner, A.I.  1983.  Pituitary adrenocortical effects on intermale agonistic behaviour.  In  "Hormones and Aggressive Behaviour",  B.B.   Svare (ed), Plenum Press, pp. 27-83.

Marsteller, F.A., Siegel, P.B. and Gross, W.B. 1980.  Agonistic behaviour and the development of the social hierarchy  in genetically diverse flocks of chickens.  Behav. Processes, 5, 339-354.

Ramenofsky, M.  1984.  Endogeneous plasma hormones and agonistic behaviour in male Japanese quail, Coturnix coturnix.  Anim. Bchav., 32, 698-708.

Rasa,  O.A.E.  and Vandenhoovel,  H.  1984.  Social stress in the fieldvole - differential  cause  of  death  in   relation  to  behaviour  and  social structure. Zeit. Tierpsychol., 65, 108-133.

Sapolsky, R.M.  1982.  The endocrine-stress-response and social status in the wild baboon. Horm. Behav., 16, 279-292.

Savory, C.J.  and MacLeod,  M.G.  1980.  Effects of grouping and isolation on feeding,  food conversion  and energy  expenditure  of domestic  chicks. Behav.  Processes, 5, 187-200.

Schuurman, T. 1980.  Hormonal correlates of agonistic behaviour in adult male rats. Prog. Brain. Res., 53, 415-420.

Serri, G.A.  and Ely,  D.L.  1984.  A comparative study of aggression related changes in brain serotonin in CBA, C57BC and DBA mice. Behav. Brain Res., 12, 283-289.

Siegel, H.S.  and Siegel, P.B.  1961.  The relationship of social competition with endocrine weights and activity in male chickens. Anim.  Behav., 9, 151-158.

Siegel, P.B. and Gross, W.B. 1973. Confinement, behaviour and performance with examples from poultry. Journ. Anim. Sci., 37, 612-617.

Siegel, H.S. and Latimer, J.W. 1975. Social interactions and antibody titres in young male chickens (gallus domesticus). Anim. Behav., 23, 323-330.

Siegel, P.B. 1976. Social behaviour of the fowl. Poult. Sci., 55, 5-13.

Siegel, H.S. 1985. Immunological responses as indicators of stress. World Poultry Sci. J., 41, 36-44.

Syme, G.J. and Syme, L.A. 1979. Social Structure in Farm Animals. Elsevier Scientific Publishing Co.

Wiepkema, P.R. and Van Adrichem, P.W.M. 1987. Biology of Stress in Farm Animals: An Integrative Approach. Martinus Nijfoff Publishers for the C.E.C.

Wingfield, J.C. and Ramenofsky, M. 1985. Testosterone and aggressive behaviour during the reproductive cycle in male birds. In "Neurobiology", R. Giles and J. Balthazart (eds), Springer-Verlag, pp. 92-104.

Wood-Gush, D.G.M. 1971. the Behaviour of the Domestic Fowl. Heinemann Studies in Biology.

Wood-Gush, D.G.M. 1983. Elements of Ethology. Chapman and Hall.

Ylander, D.M. and Craig, J.V. 1980. Inhibition of agonistic acts between domestic hens by a dominant third party. Applied Anim. Ethol., 6, 63-69.

Zayan, R. 1985. Social Space for Domestic Animals. Martinus Nijhoff Publishers for the C.E.C.

Zayan, R. 1987a. Individual recognition associated to agonistic encounters in laying hens. In "Cognitive Aspects of Social Behaviour in the Domestic Fowl", R. Zayan and I.J.H. Duncan (eds), Elsevier Scientific Publishing Co, pp. 322-438.

Zayan, R. 1987b. Spatial indicators of individual recognition in laying hens. In "Cognitive Aspects of Social Behaviour in the Domestic Fowl", R. Zayan and I.J.H. Duncan (eds), Elsevier Scientific Publishing Co, pp. 439-492.

Zayan, R. and Doyen, J. 1985. Spacing patterns of laying hens at different densities in battery cages. In "Social Space for Domestic Animals", R. Zayan (ed), pp. 37-70.

Zayan, R. and Thinès, G. 1984. Individual recognition reducing social stress in piglets grouped for the start of the fattening period. In "Results of Pig Research", (Ed IRSIA-IWONL), pp. 169-180.

Zayan, R., Doyen, J. and Duncan, I.J.H. 1983. Social and space requirements for hens in battery cages. In "Farm Animal Housing and Welfare", S.H. Baxter, M.R. Baxter and J.A.D. Mac Cormack (eds), Martinus Nijhoff Publishers for the C.E.C, pp. 67-90.

SESSION II : STIMULUS ASPECTS

# STRESS IN AGONISTIC CONTEXTS IN RODENTS

P. F. Brain

Biomedical and Physiological Research Group,
Biological Sciences,
University College of Swansea,
Singleton Park,
Swansea.
SA2 8PP
United Kingdom

## ABSTRACT

Studies assessing the endocrine consequences of exposure to fighting in rodents are briefly reviewed. 'Social stress' changes titres of many hormones with a complex time course (acute exposures to attack followed by recovery often produce quite different patterns from continuous group-housing with development of stable social relationships). Many factors e.g. species, strain, age and prior experience determine the precise responses to agonistic encounters. Some of the detrimental consequences of fighting are listed. Evidence is presented that a moderate duration of individual housing is <u>not</u> stressful in rodents but generates reactive animals. It is argued that, although agonistic contexts are a potent source of social stress, the effects are relatively transient and can be controlled.

## INTRODUCTION

It is often assumed that agonistic behaviour, especially that of males, is a potent source of stress in many species reducing weight gain, disease resistance and reproductive activity. There is, indeed, evidence that such 'social stressors' can have profound effects on the physiology and behaviour of many vertebrate species (see the volume edited by Eleftheriou and Scott, 1971). Although there is <u>no</u> simple relationship between fighting and 'stress' in the sense used by Christian (1956), it is intended to briefly review what is known of the physiological repercussions of fighting (or being subject to defeat) in male rodents and then to emphasize some of the complications that have been recently identified in this area. It is appreciated that this older material places too great an emphasis on fighting, accounts for a minor percentage of total behaviour and exclusively looks at the male (c.f. Brain, 1988a) but it seems a suitable starting point. The account certainly should be

useful in assessing the likely impact of social stress in a variety of
farm animals as they are often crowed in single sex groups.


A BRIEF REVIEW OF THE ENDOCRINE CORRELATES OF FIGHTING OR BEING SUBJECT
TO DEFEAT.

One should firstly emphasize that the view that 'stress' may be
simply reflected in the levels of generated glucocorticoids is an over-
simplification. 'Stress' is a nebulous concept and stressors can have
wide-ranging effects on a variety of endocrine (von zur Muhlen et al.
1976) and other systems. This section will briefly review what is known
about the impact of fighting on the output of particular hormones, as
these are often used as indicators of 'stress'.


## Hypothalamic factors

There has been some enthusiasm for relating hypothalamic releasing
factors to behaviour because these compounds seem intimately related to
neural functioning. Eleftheriou and Church (1968) demonstrated that
subjecting male mice to short bouts of defeat by aggressive 'trained
fighters' depressed hypothalamic luteinizing hormone-releasing factor
(LH-RF). Somewhat in contrast, Vescovi et al. (1985) recorded that both
dominant and subordinate mice (housed in pairs with social conflict) had
higher levels of this factor in the hypothalamus than undisturbed
individually-housed counterparts. Using a comparable design, Mainardi et
al. (1984) also found that hypothalamic thyrotropin-releasing hormone was
elevated in the socially experienced paired mice.


## Anterior pituitary hormones

Anterior pituitary hormones can be regarded as good indicators of
the activity of major sections of the endocrine system. Eleftheriou et
al. (1986) showed that short bouts of attack by 'trained fighters'
increased pituitary and plasma levels of thyroid stimulating hormone.
Similar intermittent exposure also elevated synthesis and release of
adrenocorticotrophic hormone (ACTH) (Bronson and Eleftheriou, 1965). It
is interesting to note with respect to ACTH, however, that rats given
electroshock who have the facility to fight generate _lower_ levels than
counterparts shocked alone. Henry and Stephens (1977) also suggested
that the glucocorticoid response to ACTH is lower in dominant mice than

in subordinates. Exposure to short daily defeats by 'trained fighters' increased serum luteinizing hormone in mice (Eleftheriou and Church, 1967; 1968) but continual exposure in pairs decreased serum follicle stimulating hormone (FSH) and LH (Bronson et al. 1973). There were few changes in pituitary levels of hormone (LH declined in dominants), in this last-mentioned study, but subordinates showed greater depressions of serum values than dominants.

## Thyroid hormones

Thyroid hormones in mammals and birds have major effects on the organism's metabolic rate. Evans and Barnett (1965/66) described how defeated wild rats show reduced thyroidal secretion and Houlihan (1963) demonstrated that crowding in voles (Microtus californicus) reduced the uptake of radio-iodine by their thyroids. More recently, Valenti and Mainardi (1988) have reviewed the association between aggressiveness in mice and thyroid hormones. When aggressive dominants confront submissive counterparts, the two categories show similar high levels of thyroxine (T4) and tri-iodo-thyronine (T3) immediately after contests. After four days of cohabitation in pairs, however, dominants have the higher hormonal titres of T3 and T4. Individually-housed subjects have levels similar to those of dominants after the establishment of stable hierarchies in the latter.

## Medullary Catecholamines

These hormones are, of course, the classical 'flight and fight' factors. Subjecting male mice to 14 brief daily defeats followed by recovery, increases medullary contents of catecholamines (it is obviously difficult to interpret such changes as the balance of synthesis and release has to be considered) compared with undefeated controls (Welch and Welch, 1969a, Goldberg and Welch, 1972). Conversely, when mice are allowed to fight vigorously for 60 minutes, they show a marked decline in adrenaline (E) content but no change in nor-adrenaline (NE) (Welch and Welch, 1969b). Gamal-el-Din (1979) found that defeated mice showed increased levels of E, whereas victors had elevated levels of NE. A single exposure to defeat produced maximal depletion of E two hours later with values returning to control levels after 24 hours. In contrast, the acute NE depletion recovered after 2 hours and was supranormal after 24 hours. When three daily defeats were employed, NE was elevated above control values 24 hours after the final encounter but E was only significantly augmented 4 days after this final experience.

Studies on the enzymes that alter catecholamines may be revealing. The adrenomedullary content of the enzyme choline acetyltransferase is elevated in defeated animals indicating increased hormonal synthesis (Welch and Welch, 1969a, Goldberg and Welch, 1972). Henry et al. (1974) demonstrated that dominant mice had elevated adrenal levels of the enzymes tyrosine hydroxylase (TH) and phenylethanolamine-N-methyl transferase (PNMT) compared with defeated counterparts. They suggested that these changes show increased synthesis of E and NE in dominants. This finding is in apparent contrast to Tizabi et al. (1976) who recorded that PNMT levels were elevated in C57BR/cdH and A/HeJ strain mice who were subjected to attack. Ely and Henry (1978) later claimed that both dominant and subordinate mice showed increased TH and PNMT after 14 days of fighting in small colonies but that subsequently (42 and 105 days after introduction) dominants consistently had higher levels of these enzymes than subordinates. Gamal-el-Din (1978) also found in acute increases in PNMT levels after fighting in both victorious and vanquished TO strain mice but, in contrast, she recorded the greater change in subordinates. A single exposure to defeat resulted in PNMT levels reaching maximal values 12 hours after the exposure to attack. Changes were more pronounced in older than younger mice. Henry and Stephens (1977) suggested that the initial fights of CBA mice in colonies are related to elevated catecholamine sympathetic arousal (associated with hypertension) whereas longer-established colonies move to elevated adrenocortical function accompanied by high PNMT levels. It is interesting in this respect to note that treatment with ACTH markedly elevates PNMT levels (Hucklebridge et al., 1981). Certainly, the time course and the age of the subjects are most important in these changes.

What then of the changes in serum concentrations of catecholamines? Hucklebridge et al. (1973) assessed plasma levels of catecholamines in mice 60 minutes after vigorous fighting. They noted that fighting increased plasma E but produced no change in NE. Naive isolates who were defeated or who fought to a 'draw' showed this increase but only 'trained fighters' in 'drawn' contests showed this phenomenon. Severe defeats elevated both E and NE. Tizabi et al. (1976) described the responses of three strains of mice from stable groups to defeat by 'trained fighter' mice. Plasma NE and E levels were determined within one minute of the last attack. Two strains (C57BR/cdJ and A/HeJ) showed greater NE and E levels after four days of attack but the third strain (NIH) only elevated elevated NE after fourteen days of attack. 'Victims' of the first two strains were allowed to recover for different periods of time after 7 days of attack exposure. Catecholamine levels in C57BR/cdJ took longer (4 days) to return to control values than the A/HeJ strain (1 day).

## Glucocorticoids

Using the procedure of short daily exposures to defeat by 'trained fighters' followed by recovery, a variety of workers (e.g. Archer, 1969; 1970; Bronson & Eleftheriou, 1964; 1965a; 1965b; 1965c; Hucklebridge et al. 1981) have shown progressively increased adrenal weight and/or elevated titres of (bound and free) corticosterone in defeated mice. Bronson and Eleftheriou (1965c) showed that the elevation of plasma corticosterone can be generated in experienced subordinates without subjecting them to physical attack by exposing them to social dominants behind a partition. Mukhammedov et al. (1976) have shown, however, that fighting disappears after 24 hours in grouped, formerly-isolated mice which is when their corticosterone levels return to baseline. Brain and Nowell (1971) reported that isolation followed by pairing produced a greater increment in adrenal weight in mice than continuous pairing or pairing followed by isolation. Although this suggests that fighting is an important factor in these adrenal changes, it did seem likely that changing the housing condition was more stressful than maintaining a particular condition. Politch and Leshner (1977) showed that the levels of corticosterone generated in attacker mice were not correlated with their amount of fighting, suggesting that the experience of defeat is crucial in such hormonal changes. Using CBA mice and stable groups, Henry and Stephens (1977) confirmed that fighting elevated plasma corticosterone but actually found greater activation in 'older' (longer-established) groups where overt fighting had declined. In their study, subordinates clearly had higher titres than dominants. A later study by Ely and Henry (1978) suggested that this distinction between dominants and subordinates disappeared 105 days after colony formation. Using more complex, presumedly-naturalistic, situations raises yet more questions.

Bishop and Chevins (1988) found, using a large, complex arena in which territories could exist, that territory holders, subdominants and subordinates did not differ in their plasma corticosterone titres or relative adrenal weights. This was true at several points of the circadian rhythm of hormonal secretion. Indeed , territory holders had higher corticosterone levels than undisturbed dominants housed in small social groups in traditional animal caging. Consequently the "stress" of maintaining a territory in competition with near neighbours may elevate plasma corticosterone levels, whereas social stability eventually allows dominants to show low titres of this hormone.

## Sex steroids

It has been known for many years that there is generally an inverse relationship between adrenocortical activity and gonadal hormone production in rodents. Substantial early reviews (e.g. Brain, 1971; Bronson, 1967; Christian, 1956; 1959; 1963a; 1963b) marshalled an impressive body of evidence (largely based on the weights of gonads and sex accessories and gland histologies) suggesting that fighting (and more especially exposure to defeat) decreased gonadal activity (and subsequent reproductive potential) Prolonged exposure to defeat (as in the long-term pairing of male mice) results in the subordinate partner having relatively suppressed preputial and seminal vesicle weights compared to its dominant cagemate (Brain, 1972; Bronson and Marsden, 1973; Lloyd, 1975). Naturally, this difference could be a consequence of defeat stress suppressing testicular androgen secretion or it could be due to the positive fighting experience in the winner stimulating such activity. More directly, McKinney and Desjardins (1973) claimed that prolonged fighting between adult male mice reduces the plasma concentration of androgens in subordinates and the capacity of their testes to synthesize this hormone in vitro. They also suggested that rearing immature males with aggressive adult males (who would be likely to expose them to defeat) suppressed spermatogenesis and plasma androgen secretion c.f. counterparts reared with docile castrates. One should note, however, that contrasting plasma testosterone levels is difficult because of the episodic release of this material. Using the complex territorial situation described earlier, Bishop and Chevins (1988) also failed to find consistent differences in plasma androgen titres in territory holders, subdominants and subordinates. Again, there was some evidence that dominant mice from small stable groups had higher plasma testosterone levels than either their subordinate cagemates or "free-range" mice. The "stress" of having to maintain a territory under such circumstances could also account for this failure.

## ADDITIONAL COMMENTS ON HOUSING CONDITIONS AND 'SOCIAL STRESS'

One should initially emphasize the ability of the House mouse to assume a wide range of social structures suited to different environmental factors (Brain, 1988a). There is consequently no obligatory social structure for this highly opportunistic species and similar flexibility may be true of some of our farm animals. This makes the interpreting of the effects of housing conditions on physiology most difficult.

As well as the data concerning hormonal responses to fighting exposure described above, there is a mass of material (recently reviewed in Brain and Benton, 1983) contrasting a variety of physiological and behavioural correlates in mice from different housing conditions. It now seems very likely that individual housing ("isolation") of male mice rather than constituting a "stress" (in terms of 'social deprivation') renders animals more aggressive because they take on the characteristics of social dominants or even territorial mice! Although individual housing naturally eliminates social conflict, it does lead to individuals becoming very reactive to novel stimuli in terms of "stress responding". Obviously considerable difficulties can be generated in some species by casually group-housing formerly individually housed males with like-sexed cagemates. There is good evidence (Brain and Benton, 1983) that precluding physical contact (rather than preventing exposure to auditory or olfactory cues) accounts for most of the behavioural and physiological consequences of individual housing. This is not to underplay the general importance of multisensorial systems in the modulation of responses to housing conditions.

Brain (1988b) has recently reviewed some of the other complexities of interpreting the literature concerned with social stress in mouse colonies. It has been emphasised that it is actually quite difficult to establish that a particular housing condition is or is not more stressful than another. It is clear that different strains of mice show varied

degrees of tolerance to group-living (see Brain, 1988a) and that their
aggressive responses can be modified by age, exposure to females, degree
of familiarity (with the housing condition and their cage-mates) and
prior (positive or negative) experience of group interactions. In mice
(as in other species) odour deposits (rather than direct attack) may have
dramatic effects on behaviour and physiology. Large arenas, sometimes
having the facility to burrow into the substrate and to construct nests,
have intrinsic appeal as they seem more naturalistic but there is little
evidence that such conditions are associated with reduced social stress.
Indeed, adult male mice are often intensely territorial under such
circumstances with prolonged attacks on resident subordinates and (more
vigorously) on intruders. Design of the cage (e.g. in the siting of
feeding and watering locations) can have a profound effects on fighting
behaviour.

Disturbance of the animals or the substrate on which they are based
generally augments fighting. One must also emphasize that although this
account has been largely limited to the kind of social aggression seen in
male mice, this species may show many forms of "aggression" expressing
differing mixes of offensive, defensive and predatory motivation (Brain,
1988a). It is by no means established that similar durations and
intensities of threat and attack in other contexts are associated with
identical "social stress".

One should finally mention that quantification of the amount of
'social stress' associated with fighting in mice is complicated by the
recent demonstration of a short-acting (up to 2 minutes) environmentally-
induced (by exposure to males or even their olfactory cues) analgesia
which is not influenced by endogenous opioids (Randall, 1988). This is
followed by a seemingly-independent, longer-lasting opioid-mediated
analgesia which can also be stimulated by attack (Randall, 1988).
Obviously, as well as complicating the time-course of "stress
responding", the degree of analgesia is likely to modify the animal's
response to attacks of similar duration and/or intensity.

DELETERIOUS EFFECTS OF 'SOCIAL STRESS'

Obviously, attack can cause tissue damage but in many species there
are behavioural mechanisms which reduce the likelihood of such injury.
As well as reducing or suppressing a defeated or subordinated mouse's

reproductive activity (there is evidence that most of the breeding is performed by dominant or territorial animals), the 'stressful' effects of fighting (and especially defeat) have other deleterious actions. Brayton and Brain (1974) have shown that "crowding" increases the retention of introduced endoparasite larvae in mice and Beden and Brain (1986a; b) have indicated that the hormonal correlates associated with 'social stress, slow the antibody response to challenge with a standard particulate antigen (sheep red blood cells). Such changes may account for the often-recorded reductions in disease resistance in defeated or subordinated rodents. The "stresses" generated by fighting may also have detrimental effects on the functioning of particular organ systems. Henry (1987) and Henry et al. (1967; 1982) have established that such stressors can produce chronic and irreversible hypertension accompanied later by arteriosclerosis and nephritis. It is interesting, in this respect, to note that Christian as early as 1963 suggested that ACTH damaged the Bowman's capsule in the kidney. Bishop and Chevins (1988) also found that blood urea levels (indicative of kidney damage) were elevated in "free range" territory holders and subordinates compared with dominants and subordinates from stable groups.

FINAL COMMENTS

Consequently the generation of social stress by fighting in mice is a complex phenomena with wide-ranging repercussions. It is really only in this species (and perhaps the rat) that some of the complexities have been examined with reasonable success. Although I have concentrated on the traditional association between hormones and fighting, other aspects of physiology should also be related to much wider descriptions of behaviour. The ethoexperimental approach is recommended here (Brain, 1989). Certainly, although the stress generated by fighting can acutely cause considerable problems leading to injury, impaired reproductive ability, failure to produce weight gain and reduced fitness in mice, there are, husbandry steps (reviewed for the mouse by Brain, 1988b) that one can take to ameliorate the effects of social conflict. One must be able to do similar things for farm animals but these would depend on the species, the strain, the age of the subjects and their prior history. One must also add that the detailed studies on rodents strongly support the conclusion that it is wrong to assume that there is a unidirectional association with 'social stress' producing hormonal changes. Hormonal variations (however produced) clearly modulate the behavioural characteristics of animals <u>and</u> change the individual's production and detection of social signals (Brain, 1989). It is hoped that the experiences gained with mice might provide insights to plan extensions of the necessary pioneering investigations on the effects of social stress in farm animals by workers such as Williams et al. (1977) on chickens and Liptrap and Raeside (1978) on pigs.

REFERENCES

Archer, J. 1969. Effects of social stimuli on the adrenal cortex in male mice. Psychon. Sci., 14, 17-18.
Archer, J. 1970. Effects of aggressive behavior on the adrenal cortex in male laboratory mice. J. Mammal., 51, 327-332.
Beden, S.N. and Brain, P.F. 1985a. The primary immune responses to sheep red blood cells in mice of differing social rank or from individual housing. IRCS Med. Sci., 13, 364-365.
Beden, S.N. and Brain, P.F. 1985b. Effects of combined castration and adrenalectomy and a variety of stressors on thymic and spleen weights and the primary immune response in mice. IRCS Med. Sci., 13, 416-417.
Bishop, M.L. and Chevins, P.F.D. 1988. Territory formation by mice under laboratory conditions: Welfare considerations. Paper presented at UFAW Symposium on "Laboratory Animal Welfare Research" (Royal Holloway and Bedford New College, London), 21st-22nd April.
Brain, P.F. 1971. The physiology of population limitation in rodents - A review. Communs. Behav. Biol. 6, 115-123.
Brain, P.F. 1972. Endocrine and behavioral differences between dominant and subordinate male house mice housed in pairs. Psychon. Sci., 28, 260-262.
Brain, P.F. 1988a. The adaptiveness of house mouse aggression. In "House Mouse Aggression: A Model for Understanding the Evolution of Social Behaviour" (Eds. P.F. Brain, D. Mainardi and S. Parmigiani). (Harwood Academic Publishers, Chur) in press.
Brain, P.F. 1988b. Social stress in laboratory mouse colonies. Paper presented at UFAW Symposium on "Laboratory Animal Welfare Research" (Royal Holloway and Bedford New College, London), 21st-22nd, April.
Brain, P.F. 1989. An ethoexperimental approach to behavioral endocrinology. In "Ethoexperimental Analysis of Behavior". (Eds. R.J. Blanchard, P.F. Brain, D.C. Blanchard and S. Parmigiani). Kluwer Academic Publishers, Dordrecht, in press.
Brain, P.F. and Benton, D. 1983. Conditions of housing, hormones and aggressive behavior. In: "Hormones and Aggressive Behavior" (Ed. B.B. Svare). (Plenum Press, New York). pp. 351-372.
Brain, P.F. and Nowell, N.W. 1971. The effect of prior housing on adrenal response to isolation/grouping in male albino mice. Psychon. Sci., 22, 183-184.
Brayton, A.R. and Brain, P.F. 1974. Effects of "crowding" on endocrine function and retention of the digenean parasite <u>Microphallus pygmaeus</u> in male and female mice. J. <u>Helminth</u>., 48, 99-106.

Bronson, F.H. 1967. Effects of social stimulation on adrenal and reproductive physiology of rodents. In "Husbandry of Laboratory Animals" (Ed. M.L. Conalty). (Academic Press, New York). pp. 513-542.

Bronson, F.H. and Eleftheriou, B.E. 1964. Chronic physiological effects of fighting in mice. Gen. Comp. Endocr., 4, 9-14.

Bronson, F.H. and Eleftheriou, B.E. 1965a. Behavioral, pituitary and adrenal correlates of controlled fighting (defeat) in mice. Physiol. Zool., 38, 406-411.

Bronson, F.H. and Eleftheriou, B.E. 1965b. Relative effects of fighting on bound and unbound corticosterone in mice. Proc. Soc. exp. Biol. Med., 118, 146-149.

Bronson, F.H. and Eleftheriou, B.E. 1965c. Adrenal response to fighting in mice: Separation of physical and psychological causes. Science (N.Y.), 147, 627-628.

Bronson, F.H. and Marsden, H.M. 1973. The preputial gland as an indicator of social dominance in male mice. Behav. Biol., 9, 625-628.

Bronson, F.H., Stetson, M.H. and Stiff, M.E. 1973. Serum FSH and LH in male mice following aggressive and non-aggressive interaction. Physiol. Behav., 10, 369-372.

Christian, J.J. 1956. Adrenal and reproductive responses to population size in mice from freely growing populations. Ecology, 37, 258-273.

Christian, J.J. 1959. The roles of endocrine and behavioral factors in the growth of mammalian populations. In "Comparative Endocrinology" (Ed. A. Gorbmann). (J. Wiley and Sons Inc., New York) pp. 71-97.

Christian, J.J. 1963a. The pathology of overpopulation. Military Med., 128, 571-603.

Christian, J.J. 1963b. Endocrine adaptive mechanisms and the physiologic regulation of population growth. In "Physiological Mammalogy" (Eds. M.V. Moyer and R.G. van Gelder). (Academic Press, New York). pp.189-353.

Eleftheriou, B.E. and Church, R.L. 1967. Effects of repeated exposure to aggression and defeat on plasma and pituitary levels of luteinizing hormone in C57BL/6J mice. Gen. Comp. Endocr., 9, 263-266.

Eleftheriou, B.E. and Church, R.L. 1968. Levels of hypothalamic luteinizing hormone - releasing factor after exposure to aggression (defeat) in C57BL/6J mice. J. Endocr., 42, 347-348.

Eleftheriou, B.E. and Scott, J.P. (Eds) 1971. "The Physiology of Aggression and Defeat" (Plenum Press, New York).

Eleftheriou, B.E., Church, R.L., Norman, R.L., Pattison, M. and Zolovick, A.J. 1968. Effect of repeated exposure to aggression and defeat on plasma and pituitary levels of thyrotrophin. Physiol. Behav., 3, 467-469.

Ely, D.L. and Henry, J.P. 1978. Neuroendocrine response patterns in dominant and subordinate mice. Horm. Behav., 10, 156-169.

Evans, C.S. and Barnett, S.A. 1965/66. Physiological effects of 'social stress' in wild rats 3. Thyroid. Neuroendocr., 1, 113-120.

Gamal-el-Din, L. 1978. Some Aspects of Adrenomedullary Function in Relation to Agonistic Behaviour in the Mouse (Mus musculus). (Ph.D. thesis Polytechnic of Central London, England).

Goldberg, A.M. and Welch, B.L. 1972. Adaptation of the adrenal medulla: sustained increase in choline acetyltransferase by psychosocial stimulation. Science (N.Y.) 178, 319-320.

Henry, J. P. 1987. Psychological factors and coronary heart disease. Holistic Med., 2, 119-132.

Henry, J.P. and Stephens, P.M. 1977. "Stress, Health and Social Environment". (Springer-Verlag, New York).

Henry, J.P., Meehan, J.P. and Stephens, P.M. 1967. The use of psychosocial stimuli to induce prolonged systolic hypertension in mice. Psychosom. Med., 33, 227-237.

Henry, J.P., Ely, D.L. and Stephens, P.M. 1974. The role of psychosocial stimilation in the pathogenesis of hypertension. Verhand. Deut. Gesell. Innere Med., 80, 1724-1740.

Henry, J.P., Meehan, J.P. and Stephens, P.M. 1982. Role of subordination in nephritis of socially-stressed mice. Clin. Exp. Hypertension, AA, 695-705.

Houlihan, R.T. 1963. The relationship of population density to endocrine and metabolic changes in the California vole Microtus californicus. Univ. Calif. Publ. Zool., 65, 327-362.

Hucklebridge, F.H., Gamal-el-Din, L. and Brain, P.F. 1981. Social status and the adrenal medulla in the house mouse (Mus musculus L). Behav. Neural. Biol., 33, 345-363.

Hucklebridge, F.H. Nowell, N.W. and Dilks,R.A. 1973. Plasma catecholamine response to fighting in the male albino mouse. Behav. Biol. 8, 785-800.

Liptrap, R.M. and Raeside, J.I. 1978. A relationship between plasma concentrations of testosterone and corticosteroids during sexual and aggressive behaviour in the boar. J. Endocr., 76, 75f-85.

Lloyd, J.A. 1975. Social behavior and hormones. In" Hormonal Correlates of Behavior". (Eds B.E. Eleftheriou and R.L. Sprott). (Plenum Press, New York). pp. 185-204.

Mainardi, M., Vescovi, P.P., Valenti, G., Martino, E. and Brain, P.F. 1984. Hypothalamic levels of thyrotropin-releasing hormone (TRH) in male albino mice of different social status. Behav. Processes, 9, 73-78.

McKinney, T.D. and Desjardins, C. 1973. Intermale stimuli and testicular function in adult and immature house mice. Biol. Reprod., 9, 370-378.

Mukhammedov, A., Nikitina, M.M. Rodinov, I.M. Rozen, V.B. and Varygin, V.N. 1976. Content of corticosterone in the blood of intact and sympathectomised animals in stress situations caused by hierarchy formation in a community of white mice. Dokl. Akad. Nauk. SSSR, 229, 223-225.

Politch, J.A. and Leshner, A.I. 1977. Relationship between plasma corticosterone levels and levels of aggressiveness in mice. Physiol. Behav., 19, 775-780.

Randall, J.I. 1988. Behavioural and Neurochemical Mechanisms of Social Conflict Analgesia in Mus musculus. (Ph.D. Thesis. Univ. of Bradford, England).

Tizabi, Y., Kopin, I.J. Maengwyn-Davies, G.D. and Thoa, N.B. 1976. Attack-induced changes in response to decapitation of plasma catecholamines of victim mice. Psychopharm. Communs, 2, 391-402.

Valenti, G. and Mainardi, M. 1988. Aggressiveness in mice and thyroid hormones. In "House Mouse Aggression: A Model for Understanding the Evolution of Social Behaviour" (Eds. P.F. Brain, D. Mainardi and S. Parmigiani). (Harwood Academic Publishers, Chur) in press.

Vescovi, P.P., Valenti, G., Mainardi, M., Brocchieri, L. and Brain, P.F. 1985. Hypothalamic levels of LHRF in male mice of differing social status and from individual housing. Behav. Processes, 11, 317-321.

von zur Muhlen, A., Dohler, D., Gartner, K and Dohler, U. 1976. Serum levels of LH, FSH, TSH, prolaectin and corticosterone in male rats after disturbance stress. Int. Endocr. Congress (Hamburg), Abstract 218.

Welch, B.L. and Welch, A.S. 1969a. Aggression and the biogenic amine neurohumors. In "Aggressive Behaviour" (Eds. S. Garattini and E.B. Sigg). (Excerpta Medica Foundation, Amsterdam). pp. 188-202.

Welch, B.L. and Welch, A.S. 1969b. Sustained effects of brief daily stress (fighting) upon brain and adrenal catecholamines and adrenal, spleen and heart weights of mice. Proc. Nat. Acad. Sci., 64, 100-107.

Williams, C.G. Siegel, P.B. and Gross, W.B. 1977. Social strife in cockerel flocks during the formation of peck rights. Appl. Anim. Ethol., 3, 35-45.

# OLFACTORY SIGNALS THAT MODULATE PIG AGGRESSIVE AND SUBMISSIVE BEHAVIOR

John J. McGlone

Department of Animal Science
Texas Tech University
Lubbock, TX 79409-2141
USA

## ABSTRACT

Social stress is common on commercial pig units at weaning of pigs and sows and during the growing period. A better understanding of olfactory communication among pigs engaged in agonistic behavior, and subsequent reduction in this harmful behavior, may lead to improvements in and animal welfare farm profits. A series of studies have examined agonistic behavior in prepuberal pigs. First, a detailed catalog of young pig agonistic behavior was collected. Individual pairs of pigs were shown to fight repeatedly before a dominance/subordinate relationship was established. Urine from fighting pigs was shown to reduce fighting among naive pigs. Urine from handled or stressed pigs was shown to increase submissive behavior. These studies lead to the hypothesis that two odor cues exist in prepuberal pigs: (A) an odor associated with fighting and dominant males that suppresses fighting among naive pigs and (B) a cortisol-dependant odor cue that increases submissive behavior and acts as a final olfactory signal of submission. Although not believed to be the prepuberal anti-aggressive pheromone, an odor of the adult boar (a dominant male) was shown to reduce aggressive behavior among prepuberal pigs. While androstenone was shown to be an effective anti-aggressive odor in prepuberal pigs, it was not effective at reducing fighting among adult sows or between adult males and females. Androstenone may act as a supernormal signal which reduces fighting among young pigs. The chemical nature of the aggressive and submissive pheromones remains a mystery.

## INTRODUCTION

Agonistic behaviors are interesting to study because they are lively behaviors of critical evolutionary importance in every vertebrate species. Further justification for study of agonistic behaviors in domestic pigs is the economic importance of harmful behaviors to animal agriculture. Additionally and outside of economics, the well being of pigs may be enhanced when social stress is minimized.

## When do pigs fight

Aggressive interactions are common when pigs are first grouped. This group-mixing induced fighting is common for the newly weaned pig, for growing pigs (at particular points in the growing period) and for newly weaned sows. It seems likely that, while there may be similarities, the mechanisms controlling sow and prepuberal pig fighting are different. Also, the mechanisms controlling chronic social stress (especially tail biting and crowding-induced social stress) might be different from the mechanisms controlling acute social stress associated with the formation of a new social hierarchy. The majority of this review concerns only the acute fighting observed as new social groups are established among prepuberal pigs.

## Consequences of agonistic behavior

Everyone who has observed pigs fight will agree that the combatants are very serious. While they only rarely kill one another, they do inflict many large wounds during the course of a battle. Pigs begin fighting within hours of birth (Hartsock and Graves, 1976). And when pigs of any age meet, a fight is a likely result.

Weight gain and feed efficiency is not altered when newly-weaned prepuberal pigs are mixed unless other stressors are present (Friend et al., 1983; McGlone and Curtis, 1985; McGlone et al., 1987a). Older growing pigs, especially those heavier than 50 kg, show a temporary set-back in weight gain after mixing (McGlone et al., 1986). In Europe, where pigs are typically limit-fed, the performance set-back due to fighting is more severe. Sherritt et al., (1974) showed that limit-fed pigs have a performance suppression associated with fighting while full-fed pigs do not show such a suppression. These results demonstrate that there is a grave negative consequence on weight gain when pigs are regrouped in the presence of another stressor. Furthermore, older pigs are capable of causing more severe injury and suppressed weight gain will be found when older pigs fight.

In addition to the wounds incurred during a battle, researchers have suggested that social stress suppressed animal health. Frank Blecha and his colleagues could not find immunosuppression among regrouped pigs in spite of evidence of a rise in plasma cortisol (Blecha et al., 1985). Thus, if fighting causes health problems in prepuberal pigs, the mechanisms have not been elucidated. The primary health concern is the wounding and subsequent skin lesions that may develop. This appears to be more of a problem on certain farms that have skin-residing opportunistic pathogens.

## VARIATION IN THE PIG-FIGHTING MODEL

Not all dyads in a newly-formed group fight and the length of each agonistic bout varies greatly among dyads. This results in tremendous variation in length and number of fights. To get an idea of the inherent variation in this behavior over time, I summarized, in table 1, the duration of fighting among control pigs over several studies. These pigs were from the same genetic stock and were observed in a standard testing procedure on different dates. More traditional model systems (for example, onset of puberty, hormone levels, etc.) have some standard level the control animals exhibit--with control animals varying perhaps 30% over time. Non-treated pigs vary by over 10-fold (or 1000%) in their level of aggression in subsequent trials. Furthermore, in single experiments, the coefficient of variation (CV) among control pigs is very high. Presented in table 1 are data from the same studies showing extreme variation within control treatments within experiments (note the CV's). In the most recent trial we ran, control pig replicate fighting ranged from zero to 20 minutes of aggressive attack over the 21-hour post-regrouping period. How can one search for ways to reduce aggression when some control pigs do not fight? At times, it seems impossible.

TABLE 1.  LEVEL OF AGGRESSIVE BEHAVIOR (MIN/21-H) FOR
CONTROL, NON-TREATED PIGS OVER SEVEN TRIALS USING AN
IDENTICAL TWO-PIG PARADIGM

| Experiment # | Aggressive Attack | | |
| | Mean | SE | CV,% |
| --- | --- | --- | --- |
| 1 | 6.20 | 2.51 | 99 |
| 2 | 8.55 | 4.01 | 115 |
| 3 | 20.31 | 8.33 | 100 |
| 4 | 5.53 | 1.69 | 75 |
| 5 | 6.93 | 3.10 | 110 |
| 6 | 1.74 | .55 | 78 |
| 7 | 5.91 | 1.87 | 77 |
| 8 | 5.53 | 1.23 | 54 |

With such extremes in variation both within control
treatments and from one study to the next, it makes
understanding this behavior very difficult.  The optimistic
view is that with such tremendous variation, the mechanisms
controlling these behaviors will be very exciting to
discover.  The natural variation in pig agonistic behavior
frustrates statisticians but excites biologists.

I intend to first summarize how pigs fight. Then,  I
examine data which attempts to dissect how odor signals
affect agonistic behavior.  Finally, I will briefly discuss
techniques which may be used to reduce the level of fighting
among newly grouped pigs.

**HOW PIGS FIGHT--THE AGONISTIC ETHOGRAM**

I recognized early that the behaviors used to describe
agonistic behavior in young pigs were very crude indeed.  In
spite of some criticism that ethograms were of little value,
I set out to describe all behaviors associated with
agonistic behavior.  By agonistic behavior I mean all the
behaviors in the continuum from threat to attack to
submission.  An excellent catalog of sow social interactions

was presented by Jensen's landmark work (Jensen, 1980 and 1982) but there was no catalog for the prepuberal pig until later (McGlone, 1985a).

The description I will relate is only for the prepuberal pig. However, many of the same behaviors are found in postpuberal pigs as well as our prepuberal model.

When pigs first meet, they investigate their environment. They will sniff and root all inanimate objects. Initially, they push and touch other pigs in ways similar to how they investigate objects in their environment. Presumably they are aware of their penmates and are making an evaluation of other pigs from a short distance. They may make a close pass at penmates with some sniffing. Later, they will more intensely sniff other pigs. Occasionally, they will walk briskly towards each other and begin attacking with little or no sniffing.

Sniffing will focus on the head with particular attention paid to the face and ears. I fully agree with Ewbank's group who suggested pigs have a functional orbital gland (near the eye) that provides information on social status (Ewbank et al., 1974). A full description of the anatomy and function of the orbital gland would help explain its role in pig social behavior.

Following (or occasionally without) a sniffing exchange, pigs assume the fighting position. Pigs face one another with their shoulders pressed together. This fighting posture has been called "facing" or "head-to-head" (McGlone, 1985a; Rushen and Pajor, 1987). Rarely, pigs start the fight at a right angle (but facing) position. The apparent objective of the pigs in this position is to place bites to the ears of their opponent. Indeed, the focus of attack is the ear bite. The winner places about three times as many bites on the ear during the fight than does the loser. Over 90% of the bites administered by the eventual winner are placed on the head, ears, neck or shoulder and 64% of the bites given are placed on the ear (McGlone,

1985a). Bites to the posterior half of the body are rare. Thus, it seems the primary bite target is the ear and ear region. Many missed ear bites land on the face, neck or shoulder.

Associated with this apparent attempt to place ear bites are some less-common behaviors. I have observed these behaviors at four research sites with four different genetic stocks. While these are less-common (compared with pigs-facing, ear bite) they are found in many fights. These less common behaviors include the head-jump and the head-under-push.

The head-jump is observed during the most intense fighting. One pig (usually the eventual winner) will place its front feet on the neck or head of its opponent and, while having this advantage, will place many ear bites. Then, a likely strategy for the pig receiving the ear bites is for it to push its head up violently, thus dislodging and sometimes flipping-over the other pig. This strategy of head-jump by one pig and head-under-push by the other pig must be viewed in slow motion to fully appreciate the events. When viewed in real time, the head-jump may not be seen nor remembered because the head-under-push is so violent. But, in slow motion, the pig performing the head-jump can be seen to inflict considerable damage to the ears.

Eventually, the fighting pigs get tired. The fight may pause. In fact 50% of the fights observed have no clear winner when four pigs are brought together all at once (table 2). These undecided fights are usually longer in duration and end probably because of sheer exhaustion. Then, that pair will fight again. In fact, in the study reported in table 2, pigs fought an average of 3.8 times (six dyads in each of ten pens showed 227 total fights). Very few (only 4%) of the fights were reversals of the original winner/loser decision.

TABLE 2. NUMBERS OF DIFFERENT TYPES OF FIGHTS SHOWN OVER A 72-H PERIOD AFTER COMBINING FOUR PIGS. DATA REPRESENT 10 GROUPS OF FOUR PIGS (OR SIX DYADS).

| Type of fight | Frequency | % |
|---------------|-----------|-----|
| Decided | 103 | 45 |
| Undecided | 113 | 50 |
| Reversal | 10 | 4 |
| Two defeat one | 1 | .4 |
| Total | 227 | |

All this means that, generally, prepuberal pigs fight twice without a winner being obvious. Then, they fight two more times (on average) and in each of these second fighting bouts, the same pig is the winner. Eventually, pigs fight and, at the end of the fight, one pig shows submissive behavior and the pair never have another overt aggressive interaction. The pair may later regulate their dominance/subordinate relationship through a subordination order (as described by Jensen, 1982 for sows).

Submissive behavior

For fights with a clear winner, the winner and loser show typical behaviors. The loser will turn its body away from the attacker. The turning-away or submissive posture is not as Rushen and Pajor (1987) described, an asymmetric parallel. The submissive pig's body is turned away from the attacker and its spine is bent so that its head and ears are turned away (see photograph 1).

The issue of what to call behaviors identified at the end of fights was raised by Rushen and Pajor (1987). They claim that pigs can not be said to be showing submissive behavior, but rather the behavior should be called defense. It is true that ear and other bites continue while the pig is in the submissive posture. But, for fights with a clear winner, the submissive posture is the last posture taken by most (if not all) prepuberal pigs in confinement.  If pigs are given more room to fight, the submissive pig may show fleeing or escape behaviors.

Rushen and Pajor's argument is simply one of semantics--what shall we call this final posture?  I prefer to call it submissive behavior and they object.  Perhaps the argument is resolved by Armin Heymer's 1977 Ethological dictionary. Heymer defines submissive behavior as "Behavior of subordinate animal in order to prevent attack; defensiveness".  Of course the submissive posture inhibits, but does not immediately stop the winning pig from biting.

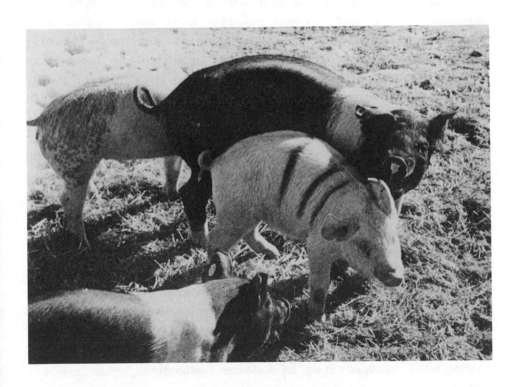

Photograph 1.  Pig attacking while smaller pig shows submissive stance.

## Repeated fights

Why pigs fight twice without a winner can best be described as exhaustion. But why pigs fight repeatedly with a clear winner is less easy to explain. If the submissive posture signals subordination, why does the winner inflict repeated wounds through repeated attacks when the submissive pig is simply giving the same visual signal? At this point, I believe the subordinate pig must give a pheromonal signal of defeat along with the visual cues before the fights stop permanently. The nature of this submissive pheromone will be discussed in the section on olfactory regulation of submissive pheromone.

## OLFACTORY SIGNALS DURING AGONISTIC BEHAVIOR

Olfactory signals are presumed to be exchanged when opponents first meet. These putative pheromones signal age, gender, physiological state and perhaps dominance status. Many excellent recent reviews should be consulted for a more broad overview of these signals (ex., Doty, 1986). My discussion will focus on the two points in the agonistic encounter that I believe olfactory information is exchanged: the start and the end of the encounter.

The sniffing that is observed among pigs upon first meeting is commonly described for many mammals. During this intense sniffing, pigs are probably assessing their probability of winning the encounter. Pigs relatively equally matched in size and physiological state will fight. Pairs of pigs in which one pig is larger or has the odor of domination (whatever that may be) may not fight because one pig immediately submits. This pre-fight olfactory assessment was the subject of a recent series of pig studies described in the aggressive pheromones section. The submissive pheromones, presumably released at the end of the fight, will be described in a later section.

## AGGRESSIVE PHEROMOMES

### Rodent aggressive pheromones

Classic rodent aggressive pheromones include those described by Mugford and Nowell (1970). They used a standard intact-male versus castrate-male paradigm for measurement of aggression. Intact male rats quickly defeated a castrated male. When urine from an intact male was painted on the fur of a castrated rat, the intact rat attacked it with greater fury. Female urine did not cause such an increased aggression. This aggressive pheromone was the odor of a male and of a dominant animal. The aggressive pheromone was not an odor produced by aggressive animals, but rather it was an odor produced by males that stimulated increased aggression. These odor cues, while interesting, would not likely be the odor cues used during agonistic encounters by fighting animals. I know of no evidence that "male odors" regulate aggressive interactions among interacting, intact males. Rather, the odors which regulate agonistic behavior should be found during agonistic interactions among animals (ex., when two males fight).

Investigations about odors which have biological importance are scarce. However, Jones and Nowell (1973) reported that odors from dominant (and more aggressive) males stimulated aggression. Other animals found this odor aversive. In the very least, these studies demonstrate that rodents can discriminate among dominant and subordinate odors and among male, female and castrate odors.

### Pig aggressive odors

Domestic pigs are known to rely heavily on their sense of smell for socially-relevant information. Meese and Baldwin (1975) showed that aggressive interactions are greatly reduced when pigs are deprived of their olfactory bulbs. Also, Ewbank et al., (1974) showed that deprivation of sight had little influence on pig aggressive behavior and establishment of a dominance order.

In 1979 I undertook a series of studies on pig aggressive pheromones under the supervision of Drs. Stan Curtis and Edwin Banks. These studies differed from the reported rodent work because I chose to examine the effects of odors produced during aggressive interactions (rather than from a particular gender). The model we chose is agriculturally-relevant. Four castrated male and female pigs were brought together in a slotted floor pen. Their behavior was observed for the first 90 minutes (when much of the fighting takes place).

The most striking and consistent finding was that urine collected from pigs while (and shortly after) engaging in an aggressive bout reduced fighting among naive test pigs (figure 1). Furthermore, urine from pigs which were handled caused an increase in total agonistic behavior. Data presented in figure 1 represent a summary of two separate studies reported in McGlone et al. (1987b). In addition to urine, pig blood plasma was also tested in another study. Plasma from only pigs that fought were tested (plasma from non-fighters was not tested) against plasma from non-regrouped pigs. Pig plasma had exactly the same effect as did urine collected from the same source. Because only plasma from aggressive pigs was tested (and if the same cue is present in the blood and urine) then the odor cue originated from the aggressive animals--and should be called an aggressive pheromone.

Urine from handled (mildly stressed) pigs increased agonistic behavior. And, because aggressive interactions are also stressful, we presumed that the handled pigs had a stress-induced odor factor that increased aggression. Fighting pigs must have that odor cue plus a far more powerful signal that reduces aggression.

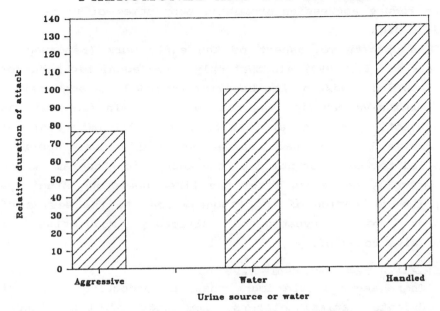

Figure 1. Relative aggressive attack is altered by painting three ml of urine on unfamiliar test pigs. Urine from handled (mildly stressed) pigs increased agonistic behavior while urine from fighting pigs reduced agonistic behavior. Distilled water was intermediate (from McGlone et al., 1987b).

In summary, two pheromones were found. One pheromone was found in the urine and blood of aggressive pigs. This pheromone reduced aggressive behavior among other pigs. The second aggressive-modulating pheromone was found in handled pigs and the second odor cue increased pig aggression.

Prepuberal males, females and castrated males all show similar levels of aggressive behavior when they are first grouped (McGlone et al., 1987). And, as found before, the aggressive-modulating pheromones were found to be present in both the castrated male and the female. However, urine from young, handled, intact males did not cause increased aggression (as did urine from handled castrate and female pigs). There remains no clear explanation for this observation--only perhaps another bit of evidence that male odors reduce aggression-promoting properties of urine from handled pigs.

An unfortunate aspect of the early work (reported in McGlone et al., 1987) was that only total agonistic behavior was recorded. Most of the behavior recorded was aggression. But submissive behavior was not recorded. In fact, it was my subjective feeling (at that time) that the nature of the aggressive behavior had changed when urine was applied. This led to the description of the agonistic ethogram (which was actually collected after the first pheromone studies). And, the collection of the ethogram lead to the series of studies which investigated olfactory modulation of submissive behavior.

Odors which modulate submission

There seems little doubt that the endocrine status of the defeated animal differs from that of the winner. Repeated throughout many species of mammals is the theme that the loser of a fight has a higher plasma glucocorticoid concentration than the winner. This higher corticoid level was found in defeated males (Fokkema et al., 1987) and females (Schuhr, 1987) compared with winning animals. In pigs, plasma cortisol rises in all animals when they are first brought together (Blecha et al., 1985) but the subordinate's plasma glucocorticoid remains higher at the end of the fight than the dominant pig's level (Arnone and Dantzer, 1980). This endocrine effect seems clear--the loser has a higher cortisol plasma concentration. The question remains, is this higher blood cortisol level reflected in an altered pheromone output (i.e., the submissive pheromone)?

I began the search for a submissive signal after observing pigs lose repeatedly, each time showing the visual sign of submission (photograph 1). I then showed that pigs who enter a fight with higher glucocorticoid level (because of an ACTH injection) are likely to lose the fight (and hence show more submission; McGlone, 1984). Then, rather than using handled pigs, I chose to use urine from ACTH-treated pigs (giving a more consistent stress simulation). I found, upon more complete behavior analyses, that urine from ACTH-treated pigs did not increase aggressive behavior, but rather such urine increased submissive behavior (McGlone, 1985b). The effect was even more pronounced when urine from ACTH-treated pigs was applied near the end of the fight (when pigs would be expected to release an olfactory signal of submission; see table 3).

TABLE 3. SUBMISSIVE BEHAVIOR (MINUTES PER FIGHT) OF PREPUBERAL PIGS WHILE URINE WAS AEROSOLIZED DURING FIGHTING BOUTS

| Treatments | | |
|---|---|---|
| Urine Type* | Time of Application | Duration of Submissive Behavior |
| Nothing | Not | $0.017^a$ |
| Saline | Early | $0.010^a$ |
| Saline | Late | $0.023^a$ |
| ACTH | Early | $0.013^a$ |
| ACTH | Late | $0.058^b$ |

*Urines collected from either saline- or ACTH-treated pigs.

These data strongly suggest the presence of a pheromone that is released during the end of a fight, that is cortisol dependant that signals submission. This could be called a "second and final signal of defeat" (after the visual signal). Existence of this second signal would explain why some fights have a clear winner (based on a visual signal) but then the pair fights again later. Theoretically, the dominance relationship could not be firm until the second signal is given and received.

100

## Biochemical nature of the submissive pheromone

We conducted a study using our late-fight urine-spraying model. In this model, urine (of various types) was sprayed on pigs while they were fighting at precisely the point at which they first show submission. If the fluid interferes with a natural odor cue, then we may say that (a) there is a natural odor cue and (b) if the level of submissive behavior is increased, then the sprayed substance adds to the effect already present.

Five treatments were tested in data presented in figure 3. When nothing was sprayed (0 ng/ml cortisol) pigs showed about 1.8 seconds of submissive behavior. When normal pig urine (from non-stressed pigs; 31 ng/ml cortisol) was sprayed, submissive behavior lasts 3.6 seconds. When urine from ACTH-treated pigs (47.8 ng/ml cortisol) was sprayed, submissive behavior lasted nearly 5 seconds. When urine was extracted with charcoal (removing most steroids and many small molecules; .7 ng/ml cortisol) or when pigs were sprayed with urine from metyrapone-fed pigs (which blocks cortisol synthesis; 17.8 ng/ml cortisol), submission was nearly as low as when nothing was sprayed. Most interesting was the high correlation between urinary cortisol[1] concentration and level of submissive behavior (r = .977; P < .001). The submissive pheromone is clearly cortisol dependent.

The final study on submissive pheromones showed statistically-similar levels of submissive behavior comparing control urine and urine spiked with cortisol. Therefore, the submissive pheromone, while cortisol dependant, is not cortisol.

---

[1]I thank Dr. Jeff Stevenson of Kansas State University for running the validated cortisol assay on these urine samples.

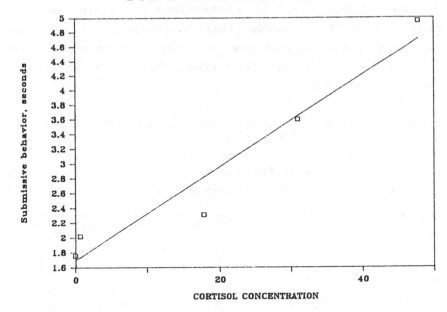

## PIG SUBMISSION BIOASSAY

Figure 2. Submissive behavior of pigs while fluids were sprayed during the late fight. X-axis is cortisol concentration of test fluids. See text for further explanation.

Supernormal odor cue

Early on in this work, we stumbled upon an anti-aggressive odor. I hypothesized that if the adult male produced odorous steroids that caused the sow to show lordosis, then these compounds must also reduce aggression. If the boar odor reduced fighting among sows the boar wanted to breed, maybe the same odor modulated young pig agonistic behavior. I was only partially correct.

The boar odor, 5-α-androst-16-en-3-one (androstenone), was found to reduce fighting among prepuberal pigs (McGlone et al., 1986; 1987a; 1988; table 4). This supernormal odor was effective in all gender combinations tested (table 5). Androstenone was not evaluated for pre-puberal boar anti-aggression. The prepuberal pig has very low, and probably not biologically-relevant concentrations of this steroid. Therefore, I must conclude that androstenone does not operate as a relevant pheromone, but rather as a super-male odor. Prepuberal pigs are less likely to attack an animal that smells like an adult.

TABLE 4.   EFFECTS OF ANDROSTENONE ON PREPUBERAL PIG
AGGRESSIVE BEHAVIOR

| Dose, µg/pig | Duration of attack[a] | | Reference |
| | Control | Androstenone | |
| --- | --- | --- | --- |
| 1000 | 20.8 | 3.7 | McGlone et al., 1988 |
| 500 | 5.9 | 2.5 | McGlone et al, 1986 |
| 5 | 20.3 | 1.8 | McGlone and Morrow, 1988 |

[a]Minutes of attack.

TABLE 5.   EFFECTS OF ANDROSTENONE ON AGONISTIC BEHAVIOR OF
PIGS OF SEVERAL GENDER COMBINATIONS

| Gender-Combination | Duration of attack | | Duration of attack | |
| | Control | Androstenone | Control | Androstenone |
| --- | --- | --- | --- | --- |
| Barrow-Barrow | 7.8 | 5.0 | 4.3 | 2.2 |
| Barrow-Gilt | 6.4 | 2.8 | 1.7 | .2 |
| Gilt-Gilt | 4.7 | 3.7 | 2.2 | .5 |
| SEM | 1.15 | | .66 | |
| Main effects of drug use | $P = .028$ | | $P = .057$ | |

It is not known to what degree androstenone modulates inter-boar aggression. But, aggressive boars did have a higher concentration of salivary androstenone than did control boars (Booth, 1980). Booth and Parrot (1986) found that steroid did not reduce fighting among sows and boars when sows were not in estrus. Finally, aggressive behavior of adult sows was not affected by androstenone spray (Stansbury et al., 1987).

In summary, androstenone has its greatest affect on the prepuberal pig. This androgen reduces aggression, but has no consistent affect on submission. Interfemale and male-female aggression are not effected by androstenone, but it is not known what influence androstenone might have on inter-boar fighting.

The anticlimax

Research aimed at understanding the mechanisms underlying pig agonistic behavior was side-tracked by the discovery of odor cues which greatly reduce the level of fighting among prepuberal pigs. We found less interest in discovering the mechanisms when we had a cure (at least for prepuberal pigs). But, perhaps if we more fully understood the underlying mechanisms, we could discover more effective preventative measures. And, there are no effective treatments available (or approved in the U.S.) to reduce fighting among sows. Subordinate post-weaned sows would find enhanced well being if they were not so thoroughly defeated (and in many cases injured) after adjusting to a new social group.

MODEL OF OLFACTORY MODULATION OF PIG AGONISTIC BEHAVIOR

When pigs first meet, they assess their opponent visually and through olfaction. Either sense (e.g., a large opponent or a dominant odor) may cause one pig to become stressed and immediately submit.

Providing the pigs are evenly matched, they begin to fight. The more skilled fighter is likely to win. Skill involves primarily placement of greater number of ear bites. Eventually, this first fight (which may be very long) ends due to exhaustion without a winner. The next fight may also be long (ex: over 5 minutes) and one pig submits, largely because he/she is tired. The next two fights have a clear winner and loser. The loser, in this common but by no means only scenario, has lost three fights. Each time he loses, he shows the submissive posture and his cortisol reaches a higher level. In the final battle, the loser has such a clear cortisol rise that the olfactory cue (the second signal of defeat) is received by the dominant pig. Interruption of the second signal (by additional stressors, for example) causes prolonged fighting because of confused signals. Crowded pigs, the model predicts, would have higher cortisol even among dominant pigs--causing revolts in the dominance order and higher levels of fighting.

The male odor (androstenone) would provide a super-dominant odor. This should cause many pigs to submit quickly thereby reducing aggression. Sedate pigs may reduce fighting because those pigs that recover more quickly from the drugs effects can take advantage of their sedated penmates. I do not know of sedative-pheromone hypothesis.

## PRACTICAL METHODS OF REDUCING AGONISTIC INJURY

I know of four efficacious methods to reduce prepuberal pig fighting: (1) do not group pigs, (2) androstenone, (3) amperozide and (4) azaperone. Figure 3 shows data from Harold Gonyou (1988; in press) from a study in which he compared the efficacy of amperozide and azaperone. Gonyou found both drugs to be effective at reducing aggressive behavior by nearly 40% (figure 3).

## DRUG EFFECTS ON AGGRESSION

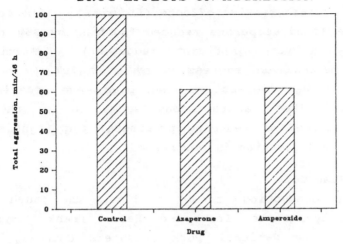

Figure 3. Azaperone and amperozide reduced relative level of pig fighting by 35 to 40% (from Gonyou et al., 1988, in press).

## DRUG AND ODOR EFFECTS ON AGGRESSION

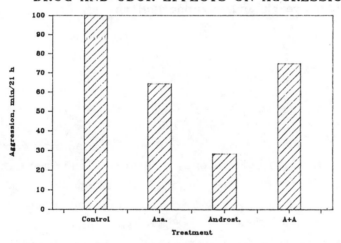

Figure 4. Relative to control pigs, azaperone reduced pig fighting by over 70%. Both drug and pheromone were as effective as azaperone alone, which indicated sedatron eliminates the odor's effect (McGlone, 1988, unpublished).

We compared azaperone, androstenone, or both drugs for their anti-aggressive effects (figure 4). Like found by Gonyou, we found azaperone reduced fighting by 35% (but in our study a non-significant reduction). Aerosolized androstenone reduced aggression by over 70% ($P = .05$). Androstenone was ineffective when pigs were sedated with azaperone. Thus, androstenone seems to be the most effective method of reducing prepuberal pig fighting. A cure for sow aggression is now needed.

## ACKNOWLEDGEMENTS

While conducting these studies, the author was supported by grants from the Harry Frank Guggenheim Foundation, the National Pork Producers Council, Humane Information Services and the state of Texas Line Item for Efficient Pork Production. Student and technical help during these studies was provided by Tom Heald, Julie Morrow, Wayne Stansbury, Bob Hurst, Eric Fugate, Chana Atkins, John Drezek and Suzanne McMinn.

## References

Arnone, M. and R. Dantzer, 1980. Does frustration induce
   aggression in pigs? Appl. Anim. Ethol. 6:351.

Blecha, F. D.S. Pollmann, and D.A. Nichols, 1985.
   Immunologic reactions of pigs regrouped at or near
   weaning. Am. J. Vet. Res. 46:1934-1937.

Booth, W.D., 1980. Endocrine and exocrine factors in the
   reproductive behaviour of the pig. Symp. zool. Soc.
   Lond. 45:289-311.

Booth, W.D. and R.F. Parrott, 1980. Body size as a
   determinant of aggression during heterosexual
   encounters in hormone-treated gonadectomized pigs.
   Aggr. Behav. 12:349-357.

Doty, R.L., 1986. Odor-guided behavior in mammals.
   Experientia. 42:257-279.

Ewbank R., G.B. Meese, and J.L. Cox, 1974. Individual
   recognition and the dominance hierarchy in the
   domesticated pig. The role of sight. Anim. Behav.
   22:473.

Fokkema, D.S., K. Smit, J. van der Gugten, and J.M.
   Koolhaas, 1987. A coherent pattern among social
   behavior, blood pressure corticosterone and
   catecholamine measures in individual male rats.
   Phsyiol. Behav. 42:485-489.

Friend T.H., D.A. Knabe, and T.B. Tanksley, Jr., 1983.
   Behavior and performance of pigs grouped by three
   different methods at weaning. J. Anim. Sci. 57:1406.

Hartsock, T.G. and H.B. Graves, 1976. Neonatal behavior and
   nutrition-related mortality in domestic swine. J.
   Anim. Sci. 42:235-241.

Heymer, A., 1977. Ethological Dictionary. Verlag Paul
   Parey, Berlin and Hamburg.

Jensen, P., 1980. An ethogram of social interaction
   patterns in group-housed dry sows. Appl. Anim. Ethol.
   6:341.

Jensen, P., 1982. An analysis of agonistic interaction
   patterns in group-housed dry sows - Aggressive
   regulation through an "avoidance order." Appl. Anim.
   Ethol. 9:47.

Jones, R.B. and N.W. Nowell, 1973. Aversive and aggression-promoting properties of urine from dominant and subordinate male mice. Anim. Learn. Behav.

McGlone, J.J., 1984. Aggressive and submissive behavior in young swine given exogenous ACTH. Domestic Animal Endocrinology 1:319-321.

McGlone, J.J., 1985a. A quantitative ethogram of aggressive and submissive behaviors in recently regrouped pigs. J. Anim. Sci. 61:559-565.

McGlone, J.J., 1985b. Olfactory cues and pig agonistic behavior: Evidence for a submissive pheromone. Physiol. Behav. 34:195-198.

McGlone, J.J., and S.E. Curtis, 1985. Behavior and performance of weanling pigs in pens equipped with hide areas. J. Anim. Sci. 60:20-24.

McGlone, J.J., 1986. Agonistic behavior in food animals: Review of research and techniquest. J. Anim. Sci. 62:1130-1139.

McGlone, J.J., W.F. Stansbury, and L.F. Tribble, 1986. Aerosolized 5α-androst-16-en-3-one reduced agonistic behavior and temporarily improved performance of growing pigs. J. Anim. Sci. 63:679-684.

McGlone, J.J., W.F. Stansbury, and L.F. Tribble, 1987a. Effects of heat and social stressors and within-pen weight variation on young pig performance and agonistic behavior. J. Anim. Sci. 65:456-462.

McGlone, J.J, S.E. Curtis, and E.M. Banks, 1987b. Evidence for aggression-modulating pheromones in prepuberal pigs. Behav. Neur. Bio. 47:27-39.

McGlone, J.J., and J.L. Morrow. 1988. Reduction of pig agonistic behavior by androstenone. J. Anim. Sci. 66:880-884.

Meese, G.B. and B.A. Baldwin, 1975. The effects of ablation of the olfactory bulbs on aggressive behavior in pigs. Appl. Anim. Ethol. 1:251.

Mugford, R.A. and N.W. Nowell, 1970. Pheromones and their effect on aggression in mice. Nature 226:967.

Rushen, J. and E. Pajor, 1987. Offence and defence in fights between young pigs (Sus scrofa). Aggr. Behav. 13:329-346.

Schuhr, B., 1987.  Social structure and plasma
       corticosterone level in female albino mice.   Physiol.
       Behav. 40:689-693.

Sherritt, G.W., H.B. Graves, J.L. Gobble and V.E. Hazlett,
       1974.   Effects of mixing pigs during the growing-
       finishing period.  J. Anim. Sci.   39:834.

Stansbury, W.F., and J.J. McGlone, 1987.   Lack of influence
       of 5α-androst-16-en-3-one (androstenone) on sow social
       behavior and post-weaning return to estrus.   Ann. Mtg.
       Amer. Soc. Anim. Sci. (Abs.).

# REACTIONS OF DAIRY CATTLE AND PIGS TO HUMANS

M. F. Seabrook
Faculty of Agricultural and Food Sciences
University of Nottingham
LE12 5RD United Kingdom

## ABSTRACT

A review of research on the interaction of humans with dairy cattle and pigs is carried out. The conclusion from this work is that the interaction between stockman and his/her animals can have a significant influence on the behaviour of animals. This conclusion is then examined in the context of social stress on animals housed in intensive environments.

## INTRODUCTION

Modern livestock production requires that the stockman, (synonymous with stockwoman, stockperson and animal caretaker), enters and imposes upon the perceived physical, social and cognitive environment of the animal. However, in most modern systems each individual stockman will have responsibility for only a small part of the production cycle, and functions in an environment where individual recognition of animals is minimised, where the number of animals dealt with is large, where the opportunity for contact with individual animals is limited and where impersonality is the order of the day.

## MAN'S EFFECT ON ANIMAL BEHAVIOUR

Metz (1987) and Seabrook (1987) have reviewed in detail the research work on the role of humans in livestock production. These reviews provide an insight into the varying role models for humans in livestock systems. These include;

Man as a RESTRAINT

Man as an OBJECT in the life space of the animal

Man in the dominance hierarchy  -as a COMPETITIVE SPECIES

-as a COMPATIBLE SPECIES

Man as an INTERACTOR with individual animals

These models can be used to suggest areas where man may significantly affect the behaviour of dairy cattle and pigs.

## Man as a restraint

Domestication of farm animals is not total as behavioural control through forced compliance and confinement is still practised. Indeed it is an essential component of modern livestock systems. Physical restraints are one of the most prevalent features of most, if not all, livestock production. Animals may thus perceive man as part of that environmental and physical constraint, in much the same way as a wall or fence. Man is thus acting as an environmental barrier. This role is highlighted at times when man is moving animals, (Grandin, 1983), when, for example, by using hands and feet man may make himself appear "bigger". However, the majority of modern livestock systems provide other even more constraining walls and barriers with man generally operating outside that wall. This is, however, not the case in less developed systems where in extensive grazing and herding systems man may indeed act as barrier, his actions setting the limits of grazing rather than using a fence, (Lott and Hart, 1979).

## Man as an object in the life space of the animal

The role of man as an environmental OBJECT is less easy to examine in isolation. Certainly animals may well prefer not to be in a particular environment and identify man in a negative way because of his presence in that environment, (Sluckin, 1979). Metz (1987) in a review of the experimental work on stockmanship concluded that many negative effects of human-animal interactions are related to the fact that the stockman induces aversive reactions and fear in their animals, simply by being in and imposing on their environment.

There are many routine husbandry practices which rely on a close approach and inspection of the animal. These include such things as, oestrus detection, supervised mating, artificial insemination, vaccinations and health inspections. There are also a number of processes, for example, castration and vaccination which involve negative stimuli. The research results show that unfamilarity with the stockman and adverse handling by the stockman can lead to physiological and behavioural responses by animals.

Man can act as a stimulator to the animal and make the environment more interesting for the animal. Dryden & Seabrook (1986) found in an experiment that sow treatments involving interaction whether, *pleasant* or *unpleasant,* resulted in piglet growth rates well above the *control.* This might suggest that it is better to have some form of interaction with the sows, even by harsh handling, than not to interact at all. The extra attention of the stockman, even in the *unpleasant* treatment, and the need for a behavioural response in a handling situation may relieve the boredom of confinement in a farrowing crate, and hence, handling provides a useful distraction from the otherwise monotonous existence of the sow. This may reduce stress on the sow and so lead to more milk for the litter.

Grandin, Curtis and Greenough (1983) showed that stimulation was important, stimulating environments were provided for a group of pigs in outdoor pens, they were given "toys" to play with. The results suggest subsequent approach to man, or, a strange object was quicker, but the animals got used to any one stimulation and needed a changing environment. A similar conclusion about stimulation is indicated by Wood-Gush and Stolba (1981).

The degree to which stimulation might affect aggression is not well defined, Carlstead (1986) showed that aggression in pigs increased when the action of the stockmen was inconsistent in the time of feeding.

## Man in the dominance hierarchy

Domestication may have required man to assume dominance over every member of the animal group, man here acting as a COMPETITIVE species. The individual animal may perceive man as an animal of another species, competing for the same territory or resources. This may be reinforced by a high level of aggression which may be an essential component of the system, (Lott and Hart, 1977), using both physical and verbal abuse.

There is little scientific information to give any insight into the perception of cattle of man, however, anecdotal material might provide some insight into the perception of man as a rival and threat, the following statements suggest the animal perceiving man in a rival role.

*"The cow attacked me as I went to pick up her calf"*
*"That bull is alright till there is a cow on heat nearby"*

Man is generally not involved in, or, imposing upon the life
space of the pig in the same way as he is with dairy cattle. However
at farrowing, and at other routine treatments, there is an imposition.

Man may be seen as the same species, or as another COMPATIBLE
species. Man in this context acting as another cow (pig etc.), an
animal to fit in the hierarchy to dominate or be dominated. The
essence of modern systems should be to create a stable environment, an
environment most closely simulating the dominance orders that appear
in nature (Wood-Gush and Stolba, 1981), creating stability and hence
less aggression, (Bartle, 1988). If man adopts the boss animal role he
may create stability more rapidly, (Seabrook, 1984).

Man may adopt the stimuli used by the animals in social
communication, for example, social grooming, (Denenberg, 1969). The
social bond so established may be important in reducing fear and in
creating a stable social hierarchy. Humans may also be able to develop
communication, for example, many nomadic husbandry systems require
communication by voice and gesture, imitating social signals, and so
exerting dominance. Modern systems with reduced space means reduced
opportunity for the animal to show signals of submission, i.e. there
is not room to move away and it may be perceived that the animal is
not in fact submitting. Man will in fact find it easy to dominate.

## Man as an interactor with individual animals
- Dairy Cattle

There is a tendency to find patterns of paradoxical behaviour in
cattle, animals tending to both initiate approach and avoidance
behaviour (Hediger, 1955). The approach behaviour is to investigate
and explore the flight behaviour to avoid contact. Flight distance may
be a measure of the animals' reaction to man, this distance varies
from herd to herd, suggesting that man is influencing it, and from
animal to animal, suggesting individual interaction between man and
animals is important. Albright (1978) indicated that higher
performance herds tended to have more approach behaviour and less
flight or avoidance behaviour.

Another measure of individual reaction effects is the time taken
for dairy cows to enter the milking parlour. Seabrook (1984) presented
results which suggested it was not a matter of design of the system

but rather the reaction of individual animals to the actions and nature of the stockman, Table 1.

TABLE 1  Behaviour differences for different stockmen and herds

| ACTION OR EVENT | Behaviour differences |
|---|---|
| Entry time to parlour | Faster for higher yielding herds |
| Field flight distance | Shorter for higher yielding herds |
| Approaches to observer | More on higher yielding herds |
| Stockman touching cows | More on higher yielding herds |
| Stockman talking to cows | More on higher yielding herds |

Seabrook (1984)

Where there is close contact between man and animals then man draws the animal into his lifespace, man thus acting as an INTERACTOR. Seabrook (1984) has shown that contact such as patting and stroking the cow is correlated with higher performance. If these are done at milking time it may encourage the cows to enter the parlour and exhibit less stress and hence less inhibition of milk let down (Albright, 1978). There are a range of interaction factors e.g. voice, gestures, smell, sound. Gonyou, Hemsworth and Barnett (1986) and others have highlighted this interaction process.

Albright (1984) when discussing training of cattle found in experiments that cattle could sometimes be slow to learn in reinforcement experiments. Using a pattern of experiments based on Krushinsky, (Albright, Kilgour and Whittlestone, 1982), it was found that cows took a long time to learn a feeding pattern when in the presence of man, but quicker if man was not there. They appeared to anticipate that man would help them out, and they became conditioned on his actions, (Albright, 1984). Sambrus and Unshelm (1983) suggest that too high a level of social bonding in farm animals is not ideal because the animal may become too dependent on man for its social interactions. It can be argued, however, there is less stress if they do relate to man. Thus the answer may be  not to isolate one animal but relate and interact with all to the same level. Seabrook (1984) highlighted confidence and consistency as being more effective in creating stability.

Animals do not function in isolation and their temprament will vary, and may be influenced by their caretakers (Stricklin and Kautz-Scanavy, 1984). A cow's fear of an aggressive handler may upset her, and one disruptive animal can unsettle a herd, (Burnside, Kowalchuk, Lambroughton and MacLeod, 1971).

- Pigs

Hemsworth, Brand and Willems (1981) found in a study of similar commercial units that sows which produced the lowest number of piglets per year displayed a greater withdrawal response to the approaching observer's hand and a lower approach behaviour towards the stationary observer. Their conclusion was that it was the relationship which developed between animal and stockman that was influencing behaviour and performance. In an attempt to investigate the relationship further Hemsworth, Barnett and Hancon (1981) studied the effect on gilts of different components of stockman behaviour, *pleasant handling* and *unpleasant handling*; they concluded that gilts in the *unpleasant handling* treatment spent less time near humans, had higher corticosteroid levels and displayed fewer interactions with the observer, they also had lower growth rates.

Dryden & Seabrook (1986) indicated that in an experiment there were significant behaviour differences between sows given *pleasant* treatment and those give *unpleasant* treatment. The *unpleasant* treatment group always showed a much greater time to come to feed when in the presence of humans than the *pleasant* treatment group, suggesting that the sows did perceive the treatments differently and indicating that the sow responds more favourably as far as approach behaviour is concerned to *pleasant* treatment, pleasant  handling improves approach behaviour and unpleasant handling makes it worse. Table 2 summarises some of research work in investigating stockman behaviour and pig behaviour effects. As well as handling, tone of voice might be important.

TABLE 2   The behaviour of the stockman and its effect on pig
behaviour and performance

| ACTION OF STOCKMAN | REACTION OF PIGS | Source | |
|---|---|---|---|
| Stroking and scratching sow's head *(pleasant)* | -the sows were less restless | Hemsworth et al | / Dryden & Seabrook |
| | -the sows were quieter | Hemsworth et al | / Dryden & Seabrook |
| | -the sows were more approachable | Hemsworth et al | / Dryden & Seabrook |
| | -larger number of piglets reared | Hemsworth et al | |
| | -some evidence of increased piglet growth rates | Dryden & Seabrook | |
| Slapping sow's head and shoulders *(unpleasant)* | -the sows were more restless | Hemsworth et al | / Dryden & Seabrook |
| | -the sows were less approachable | Hemsworth et al | / Dryden & Seabrook |
| | -reduced sexual development | Hemsworth et al | |
| | -higher corticosteroid levels | Hemsworth et al | |

Hemsworth, Brand and Willems (1981)
Hemsworth, Barnett and Hansen (1981)
Dryden and Seabrook (1986)


Some of the reactions observed may involve man as a trainer,
Lebatteux (1987). By operant conditioning the stockman may make the
animal submissive and hence dominated. For example, if the stockman
rewards behaviour of the pigs which is considered desirable, by
contact or hand feeding them a little food, the pigs will learn to
adopt that behaviour.

A number of signals intentionally or unintentionally released by
the stockman when attempting to impose routines may be identified by
the animal as threatening in nature, and so delay or interfere with
the development of a good relationship. The importance of this
relationship and the correct behaviour of the stockman in order to
create a good relationship have been demonstrated by a number of
research workers and man's active role has implications for the study
of social stress.

THE IMPLICATIONS FOR SOCIAL STRESS

Evidence that man has an effect on behaviour has been shown by numerous research workers and in addition to the summary in this paper both Seabrook (1987) and Metz (1987) have reviewed the work. The conclusion from the work is that man can influence animal behaviour in significant ways. Indeed it could be argued that in intensive livestock systems it is not possible to consider animal behaviour in isolation from the behaviour of the stockman. For example, Dryden and Seabrook (1986) have shown that "pleasant" handling of sows alters their behaviour. In this work the sows' behaviour was observed at random times during both day and night, at the entry of the observer. The general response was varied but it did appear to depend on the treatment. The "pleasant" treatment group showed some change with some sows slowly getting up with some quiet grunting, appearing to welcome man by standing, or, sitting up slowly into a more accesible position for contact. The "unpleasant" treatment group behaved very differently; standing or sitting quickly and violently with loud grunting. The sows in the "unpleasant" treatment appeared very restless, preparing either to fight or run away, and generally were more difficult to deal with. Man is thus having an effect by his actions. Hemsworth, Barnett and Hansen (1981) suggest that "pleasant" treatment gives less adrenalin release, less stress and more rest. Similarly Metz (1987) reinforces the importance of the adaption of the animal to humans, procedures like early handling and "gentling", in other words stroking, may help the animals to cope with stressful conditions. Dantzer and Mormède (1983) emphasise differences between species and individuals of the same species, so all may not be able to cope, i.e. there are considerable differences between individual animals and so the stockman should be able to interpret the individual reactions of their animals, in order to judge the correct behaviour to adopt. This sensitivity can to some extent be learned.

Metz (1987) also suggests that habituation can diminish the negative effects of restraint and that habituation is likely to occur only when the stockman frequently interacts positively with his animals. This occurs at milking and other regular routines. Metz (1987) indicates that early grooming of new born calves induced some stress. Fear may be reduced by frequent handling rather than prolonged handling.

The logical conclusion from this is that in order to reduce the stress created by an intensive system, stockmen should adopt the correct mode of action. Stress would appear to be influenced by the stockman and a positive interaction between man and animal seems desirable. Table 3 summarises the factors associated with creating a good relationship between stockman and animals.

TABLE 3   Factors associated with the development of a good relationship between man and animal.

| FACTOR IN THE RELATIONSHIP | ACTION OF THE STOCKMAN |
|---|---|
| PHYSICAL CONTACT | stroking, scratching head and patting |
| SOCIAL IDENTIFICATION WITH THE ANIMALS | use of voice and social gestures |
| CREATING A STABLE ENVIRONMENT | consistent and confident actions |
| OBSERVATION OF ANIMALS | effective development of perceptual skills |

CONCLUSION

If the scenario that man has a significant effect on animal behaviour is accepted then a number of issues pose themselves;

a. Should all stockmen have to have a licence and be tested on their relationship with stock ? A licence to care for stock would only be given if they could produce a good relationship.

b. Should this licence be given only for a limited period and then further testing takes place ?

c. Is it possible to lay down effective relationship and stockman behaviour guide lines for each species ?

d. Are we asking the stockman to attempt to ameliorate unacceptable systems? In other words, has an animal which is devoid of an environment where it can express a behaviour, such as turning round, but is treated "pleasantly" by the stockman, had a real improvement in its welfare status ?

e. Can the routine use of tranquilisers, sedatives or other behaviour modifying drugs ever be   justified on the grounds of "improved animal welfare" ? Instead attempts should be made to deal with the causes and not merely to treat the symptoms. This may mean designing systems that; minimise the mixing of unfamiliar animals,   which avoid excessive animal confinement and have positive levels of human/animal interaction.

If there is a move to  "better" animal welfare systems it must be recognised that the success of these depends a great deal on the skill of the stockman particularly his/her perceptual skills. Seabrook (1987) has reviewed these skills.

REFERENCES

Albright, J.L. 1978. The behaviour and management of high yielding dairy cows. BOCM Silcock Dairy Conference, London.
Albright, J.L., Kilgour, R. and Whittlestone, W.G. 1982. The Krushinsky Apparatus: A test for self-awareness in farm animals. Indiana Acad. Sci., 91, 595-596.
Albright, J.L. 1984. Human-animal interaction. Symposium 1, Applied Ethology Meeting, University of Carbondale, Illanois.
Bartle, N. 1988. Aggression levels in mixing dry sows. University of Nottingham Report (in print).
Burnside, E.B., Kowalchuk, W.B., Lambroughton, D.B. and MacLeod, N.M. 1971 Canadian cow dispersals. Can. J. of Anim. Sci., 51, 75-78.
Carlstead, K. 1986. Predictability of feeding: its effect on agonistic behaviour and growth in grower pigs. Appl. Anim. Behav. Sci., 16, 25-38.
Dantzer, R. and Mormède, P. 1983. Stress in farm animals; a need for a re-evaluation. J. of Anim. Sci., 57, 6-18.
Denenberg, V.H. 1969. The effects of early experience. In "The behaviour of domestic animals". (Ed. E.S.E. Hafez). (Bailière, Tindall and Cassell, London). pp 95-130.
Dryden, A.L. and Seabrook, M.F. 1986. An investigation into some components of the behaviour of the pigstockman and their influence on pig behaviour and performance. J. of Agric. Manpower Soc. 1(12), 44-52.
Gonyou, H.W., Hemsworth, P.H. and Barnett, J.L. 1986. Effects of frequent interactions with humans on pigs. Appl. Anim. Behav. Sci., 16, 269-278.
Grandin, T. 1983. Welfare designs of handling facilities. In "Farm animal housing and welfare". (Ed. S.H. Baxter, M.R. Baxter and J.A.C. MacCormack). (Nijhoff, The Hague). pp 137-149.
Grandin, T., Curtis, S.E. and Greenough, W.T. 1983. Effects of rearing environment on the behaviour of young pigs. J. of Anim. Sci., 57, 137 (abs).
Hediger, H. 1955. Studies of the psychology and behaviour of captive animals in zoos and circuses. (Criterion Books, New York).

120

Hemsworth, P.H., Brand, A. and Willems P. 1981. The behavioural
    response of sows to the presence of human beings and its
    relation to productivity. Livest. Prod. Sci.
    8, 64-74.
Hemsworth, P.H., Barnett, J.L. and Hansen, C. 1981. The influence of
    handling by humans on the behaviour, growth and corticosteroids in
    the juvenile female pig. Hormones and Behav. 15, 396-403.
Lebatteux, B. 1987. Training in the specific skills required by the
    stockman. In "The role of the  stockman in livestock productivity
    and management" (Ed. M.F. Seabrook).  (C.E.C. Luxembourg). pp107-
    117.
Lott, D.F. and Hart, B.L. 1977. Aggressive domination of cattle by
    Fulani herdsmen and its relation to aggression in Fulani culture
    and personality. Ethos, 2, 174-186.
Lott, D.F. and Hart, B.L. 1979. Applied ethology in a nomadic cattle
    culture. Appl. Anim. Ethol., 5, 309-319.
Metz, J.H.M. 1987. The response of farm animals to humans - examples of
    the epistemology of experimental research. In "The role of the
    stockman in livestock productivity and management"
    (Ed. M.F. Seabrook).  (C.E.C. Luxembourg). pp23-37.
Sambrus, H.H. and Unshelm, J. 1983. Influence of man on behaviour and
    production of animals. Proc. EAAP meeting, Madrid.
Seabrook, M.F. 1984. The psychological interaction between the stockman
    and his animals and its influence on performance of pigs and dairy
    cows. Vet. Rec. 115, 84-87.
Seabrook, M.F. 1987. The role of the stockman in livestock productivity
    and management; Research  epistemology - the holistic approach. In
    "The role of the stockman in livestock productivity and management"
    (Ed. M.F. Seabrook).  (C.E.C. Luxembourg), pp39-51.
Sluckin, W. 1979. Fear in animals. (Van Nostrand Reinhold, London).
Stricklin, W.R. and Kautz-Scanavy, C.C. 1984. The role of behavior in
    cattle production. Appl. Anim. Ethol., 11, 359-390.
Wood-Gush, D.G.M. and Stolba, A. 1981. Pig behaviour. Farmers Weekly,
    March 13, pp96-100.

REACTIONS OF POULTRY TO HUMAN BEINGS

Ian J.H. Duncan

AFRC Institute of Animal Physiology & Genetics Research,
Edinburgh Research Station, Roslin,
Midlothian EH25 9PS, Scotland

ABSTRACT

The dominant reaction of the progenitors of domestic poultry species
to human beings is a fearful one which may have been attenuated but is
unlikely to have been eliminated by the domestication process. The
behavioural responses of domestic fowl to an approaching human being are
looking around, cessation of current behaviour, orienting away, moving
away and finally crouching or escape. Heart rate rises through this
sequence to a very high level when birds are caught. There are strain
differences in intensity of response. These reactions are resistant to
modification in adult birds but may be ameliorated in young birds by
imprinting, habituation or reciprocal inhibition. Since fear is a state
of suffering which reduces welfare, the problem of fear caused by human
contact requires a solution. This may be achieved either by genetic
means or by developing techniques based on habituation or reciprocal
inhibition and applying them to the birds when they are at
a susceptible age.

INTRODUCTION

Although there is a large body of knowledge on the behaviour of
domestic animals and particularly on the behaviour of poultry, relatively
little information is available on the reactions of domestic animals to
human beings. This is partly a consequence of the direct transfer to
applied studies of the 'ethological method', whereby every effort is made
to reduce or eliminate the 'human observer effect'. While this is a
commendable aim, it has led to a tendency to eliminate the effects of
human beings from applied behavioural studies entirely. The paucity of
information in this area is now retarding progress in animal welfare
studies, since the interaction of man with animal is one of the main
causes of reduced welfare (Duncan, 1974; Wood-Gush et al., 1975;
Hemsworth and Barnett, 1987).

EVOLUTIONARY CONSIDERATIONS

An understanding of the reactions of poultry to human beings
requires some consideration of the evolutionary history of the species
involved. The species to be considered here are the common agricultural
avian species, namely the domestic fowl, turkey, duck and goose, and it

should be said that very little information is available on the early history of any of these species. Perhaps the most obvious point to be made is that the modern wild species, which are thought to share common ancestry with the domestic species, that is junglefowl (<u>Gallus gallus spp.</u>), wild turkey (<u>Meleagris gallopavo</u>), mallard duck (<u>Anas platyrhynchos</u>), muscovy duck (<u>Cairina moschata</u>), greylag goose (<u>Anser anser</u>) and swan goose (<u>Anser cygnoides</u>), all serve as prey species to man in various parts of the world today. There can be little doubt, then, that the original relationship between human beings and the progenitors of poultry was a predator-prey one. In any relationship of this sort, one would expect the dominant reaction of the prey species to the predator to be a fearful one, as has been pointed out by Gray (1971). He observed that stimuli which signal 'special evolutionary dangers' are one class of stimuli which will lead to a state of fear. In the case of the poultry species, the dangers will be those associated with predators (Duncan, 1985). Of course the process of domestication, which involves taming, or the reduction of the flight distance to human beings (Hale, 1969), will have reduced this fear of human beings as predators. Also, Craig (1981) has suggested that domestication is usually accompanied by an increase in placidity, and this might mean a reduction of general fearfulness. However, Craig (1981) also states that some breeds of domestic fowl, which have been selected for fighting ability for many generations (Wood-Gush, 1959), may be exceptions to this general rule.

An example of a difference in fearfulness between a domestic species and its putative ancestor was reported by Desforges and Wood-Gush (1975). They compared the reactions of Aylesbury and mallard ducks to a variety of stimuli including human beings. Both groups of ducks had been hatched in an incubator, artificially reared and similarly exposed to human beings. In tests involving escape from a human handler, mallards ran away significantly faster than Aylesburys. In other tests, the Aylesburys habituated faster to a stuffed model hen, novel food and a novel food container than did mallards. The decreased fear of human beings of the domestic species, therefore, may have been specific, may have been part of a general reduction in fearfulness or may have been due to a combination of two such processes accompanying domestication. What should be emphasized is that the differences were mainly of degree and not of quality.

It should also be underlined that fear of human beings is not a learnt response. Murphy and Duncan (1978) reported that domestic fowl of two stocks, which had been reared with no human contact for the first six weeks of their lives, showed fear responses on the first occasion on which they saw a human being.

In summary then, the dominant reaction of the progenitors of domestic poultry species to human beings is a fearful one which may have been attenuated but is unlikely to have been eliminated by the domestication process.

## EXPERIMENTAL EVIDENCE ON THE REACTIONS OF POULTRY TO HUMAN BEINGS

The division of this section into 'fundamental' and 'applied' studies is somewhat artificial. In general, studies aimed at elucidating the inherent nature of the reaction of poultry to human beings have been placed in the former category and those aimed at solving particular husbandry problems have been placed in the latter. There is, of course, much overlap.

### Results from fundamental studies

In a wide-ranging study of fear in domestic fowl, Murphy (1976) showed that a stock generally considered to be 'flighty' showed much more avoidance of human beings than one considered to be 'docile'. This difference could not be wholly explained in terms of greater general fearfulness, since, although the flighty birds also showed more fear in strange environments (Murphy and Wood-Gush, 1978), they showed less fear of novel foods and novel objects than did docile birds (Murphy, 1977). This difference between these two types of bird was nicely demonstrated in an experiment by Jones et al. (1981). The behavioural and physiological responses of individual hens of the two types of bird to a slowly approaching human being were recorded while they were feeding. The sequence of behavioural changes included looking around, ceasing feeding, withdrawing from the front of the cage, orienting away, and finally crouching or escape. Heart rate, as measured by radiotelemetry, rose from a mean level of 303 beats/min when the birds were at rest, to 465 beats/min when the cage was opened and the bird caught and held at the conclusion of the approach. The behavioural and physiological changes had similar time courses which supported the concept of fear

being an intervening variable having simultaneous effects on heart rate
and behaviour.    There were also differences in response between the
strains which confirmed Murphy's (1976) earlier findings.    At the start
of each observation, food was presented in a novel way and the docile
strain showed more fear of this than did the flighty strain.    Also, when
the human being was far from the birds (25-30 m) and perhaps not
recognized as a human being but only as a strange object, the docile
strain showed more signs of low level fear than did the flighty strain.
However, when the human being was close to the cage, the flighty strain
showed higher indices of fear.

## Results from applied studies

The reaction of poultry to human beings has assumed new importance
with the realization that events connected with catching and transporting
poultry are amongst the most stressful that they experience (Gerrits et
al., 1985).    Duncan et al. (1986) compared the stressfulness of
harvesting broiler chickens in a large flock by hand and by machine.    The
manual method was the traditional technique of catching the birds by
hand, inverting them and carrying them by one leg in a group of 5 over a
short distance.    The machine moved slowly towards the flock and birds
were picked up by two counter-rotating rotors fitted with soft rubber
fingers and deposited on a sloping conveyor belt which moved them to the
rear of the machine.    The heart rate of a sample of birds was measured as
they were harvested using radiotelemetry techniques.    The heart rate of
birds caught by both methods rose to similar high values but that of
birds caught by machine returned to near normal rates more quickly,
suggesting that they were less frightened.    Another sample of birds were
tested for fearfulness by the tonic immobility test immediately after
harvesting.    The duration of tonic immobility was much longer in
manually-caught birds.    These results suggest that stress could be
reduced and welfare improved by catching and picking up broiler chickens
by a carefully designed machine, rather than by hand.

A series of experiments was subsequently carried out to simulate the
catching and crating of broilers in the laboratory with a view to
identifying the most stressful components (Kite and Duncan, in
preparation).    A battery of indices of stress or disturbance were used
(wherever possible in combination) including plasma corticosterone level,

heart rate change, heterophil/lymphocyte ratio, duration of tonic immobility and latencies to resume feeding, drinking and social contact. In one of the experiments, four treatments involving varying degrees of human contact were compared. The treatments were (a) approach by the experimenter, (b) approach plus restraint by the experimenter, (c) approach plus restraint plus lifting off the ground by the experimenter and (d) restraint by the unseen experimenter. The results of the behavioural tests, particularly the latency to feed test, showed that there was a trend, with human approach causing the least response and concealed restraint causing the greatest response with the other two treatments intermediate. The large response to the concealed restraint could be explained by the extreme novelty of this situation. The heart rate response was much less variable. All the treatments caused an increase of about 70 beats/min above the baseline of about 320 beats/min. Other experiments confirmed that the most stressful aspect of the harvesting process is the catching/restraining component. It was shown that this was less distressing when it was carried out as quickly as possible and in the dark compared with in the light. It is now thought that one of the advantages of the harvesting machine is that it restrains the birds for a very short time.

## ATTEMPTS TO MODIFY THE REACTIONS OF DOMESTIC FOWL TO HUMAN BEINGS

There have been several attempts to modify the fearful reactions of domestic fowl towards human beings. There would seem to be three mechanisms by which this could be accomplished - imprinting, habituation and reciprocal inhibition.

### Imprinting

Although there can be little doubt that fear reactions can be reduced by imprinting young chicks to a human figure (consider the well-known photographs of Konrad Lorenz with goslings in train), it has never been considered seriously as a practical solution to the problem of fearfulness in poultry because of the labour required and because it might result in too much attraction to human beings.

### Habituation

Habituation is a simple form of learning whereby repeated

applications of a stimulus result in decreased responsiveness. Techniques which undoubtedly involve habituation have been used with poultry although they have often been called something else. The procedure called 'handling' has received some attention from poultry scientists following reports that handling of laboratory rats early in life led to increased growth rates (Ruegamer et al., 1954; Weininger, 1956). There is evidence that handling of domestic fowl, which have had a 'normal' amount of contact with human beings, is fear-inducing and stressful (Hughes and Black, 1976; Murphy and Duncan, 1977; Beuving 1980; Jones et al., 1981). Research which looked at the effects of repeated handling has produced conflicting results. It should be said, however, that the level of fearfulness after handling has seldom been measured directly and this makes the interpretation of these results rather tentative. Freeman and Manning (1979) found that regular handling of chicks of a layer strain decreased growth rate, suggestive of a stressful effect and of no habituation to human beings. McPherson et al. (1961) working with broilers to 8 weeks, and Reichman et al. (1978), working with broilers to 5 weeks and laying pullets to 31 weeks of age, found that frequency of handling had no effect on growth rate. On the other hand, Thompson (1976) obtained increased growth in broilers following early handling. Also, Jones and Hughes (1981) found enhanced growth in broilers and in the females but not the males of two layer strains following regular handling from hatching to 3 weeks of age. Moreover, Gross and Siegel (1979) reported that immature males of a laying strain grew faster and habituated behaviourally to a short daily period of adaptation to their handler. In a study which looked more directly at fear responses, Jones and Faure (1981) showed that regular handling of three strains of chicks over the first 5 weeks of life decreased tonic immobility, a fear-potentiated phenomenon, and increased approach to a human being, but had no effect on approach to an inanimate object. Jones and Faure (1981) concluded that handling does not depress general fearfulness, but specifically reduces fear of human beings, presumably through habituation.

Unfortunately, in none of these studies was a control treatment included in which the birds had no human contact at all. Thus it is impossible to tell whether the increased growth rates described in three of these reports is due to habituation alone or to some additional stimulating property of handling. With regard to the apparent conflicting evidence on handling, it should be said that slight differences in procedure can probably account for major differences in results. For example, one would expect faster habituation if the handling was regular, frequent, gentle and occurred early in the bird's life.

There has been one experiment carried out in which the reactions of birds to human beings was recorded after the birds had been reared with no human contact at all (Murphy and Duncan, 1978). Chicks of the flighty and docile strains, which had been reared with no human contact for the first 6 weeks of their lives, showed withdrawal responses when first they were exposed to human beings. Chicks of the flighty strain showed more withdrawal than those of the docile strain. However, whereas the docile birds habituated quickly to human beings and after 5 days were responding in the same way as control docile birds which had been reared with normal human contact, the flighty birds were still showing more withdrawal than their controls after 21 days. These results suggest that the great difference in response to human beings between adult birds of these two strains is partly a genetically determined difference in withdrawal response present from hatching and partly a difference in learning, birds of the docile strain showing more habituation of withdrawal than those of the flighty strain.

There has been some debate in the scientific literature on the effects of human presence and handling where this is incidental to the main aims of experiments on fear. For example, some studies have found that human presence increases fear in chicks as measured by the tonic immobility test (Gallup et al., 1972; Gallup, 1977) and open-field test (Gallup and Suarez, 1980; Suarez and Gallup, 1982). On the other hand, Jones (1987) found no effect of human presence on the behaviour of chicks in an open-field. Once again, these discrepant results can probably be explained in terms of slight differences in procedure. Moreover, one could imagine that human contact might add to the level of fear if the birds were not accustomed to human beings, but actually have the opposite effect (by providing familiar cues in a very strange environment) if the birds were well habituated to them.

## Reciprocal inhibition

Reciprocal inhibition is the process whereby arousal of the parasympathetic nervous system tends to inhibit activity in the sympathetic nervous system. It has been used by psychotherapists to overcome irrational fears in patients (Wolpe, 1958). Murphy and Duncan (1978) attempted to use this technique to modify the fear responses of domestic fowl towards human beings. A food reward was associated with human contact on 6 consecutive days. The responses of adult hens of the flighty and docile strains to human beings were very resistant to modification. It is of interest that the birds showed habituation to other aspects of the experimental procedure (by starting to eat more quickly and by eating more as the experiment proceeded), suggesting that the lack of change to human beings was very specific. On the other hand, the results from a similar experiment, which used chicks of the same two strains, suggested that their responses were more easily modified. The association of human contact with a food reward resulted in chicks of the docile strain showing an increased amount of approach towards a human being. However, this same association had no effect on the withdrawal responses of chicks of the flighty strain.

## PRACTICAL IMPLICATIONS

The evidence presented in this paper indicates that the dominant reactions of poultry to human beings are fearful. In itself fear is a state of suffering which reduces welfare (Duncan, 1987) and which, therefore, should be eliminated or reduced. In addition, some of the responses made by the birds may be so violent that they lead to injury and a further reduction in welfare. At the present time, some human contact is unavoidable. The human contact made with chicks shortly after hatching as they are moved to brooders is unlikely to frighten them, since fear of visual stimuli takes a few days to develop (Duncan, 1985). Thereafter most husbandry procedures can now be carried out automatically. The exceptions are (in the case of laying stock), when the birds have to be moved from brooders to rearing quarters and from there to the laying environment. Even when this happens within the same cages, a certain amount of dispersion, including human handling, is necessary. Again, at the end of their lives, all birds have to be moved from their living quarters to a place of slaughter, and this usually involves a lot of human contact. Moreover, most European welfare laws or welfare codes insist that all birds are visually inspected every day, and this is not possible, or more correctly, not feasible at present without a human being coming close to the birds. Furthermore, all these necessary contacts with human beings are likely to become more traumatic to the birds as increasing automation reduces the opportunities for habituation to occur.

What can be done to alleviate the situation? One possibility may be in genetic selection of birds that are less fearful of human beings. Faure (1980) has discussed the feasibility of doing this with regard to general fearfulness and, if the breeding companies were sufficiently motivated, this would certainly seem to be a possibility. In fact, some egg producers have achieved an improvement based on genetics when they have switched to using certain placid brown egg laying strains. the other solution would seem to lie in developing techniques based on habituation or reciprocal inhibition. This development would be speeded up if the stimulus properties of human beings which cause fear could be identified. It might then be possible to design a model with these properties which could be presented automatically and regularly to the birds at their most susceptible age, perhaps in conjunction with food delivery.

REFERENCES

Beuving, G. 1980. Corticosteroids in laying hens. In "The Laying Hen and Its Environment" (Ed. R. Moss). (Martinus Nijhoff, The Hague). pp. 65–84.
Craig, J.V. 1981. Domestic Animal Behavior. (Prentice Hall, New Jersey).
Desforges, M.F. and Wood-Gush, D.G.M. 1975. A behavioural comparison of domestic and mallard ducks. Habituation and flight reactions. Anim. Behav., 23, 692–697.
Duncan, I.J.H. 1974. A scientific assessment of welfare. Proc. Br. Soc. Anim. Prod., 3, 9–19.
Duncan, I.J.H. 1985. How do fearful birds respond? In "Second European Symposium on Poultry Welfare" (Ed. R.-M. Wegner). (German Branch of the W.P.S.A., Celle). pp. 96–106.
Duncan, I.J.H. 1987. The welfare of farm animals: an ethological approach. Sci. Prog. Oxf., 71, 317–326.
Duncan, I.J.H., Slee, G.S., Kettlewell, P., Berry, P. and Carlisle, A.J. 1986. Comparison of the stressfulness of harvesting broiler chickens by machine and by hand. Br. Poult. Sci., 27, 109–114.
Faure, J.M. 1980. To adapt the environemnt to the bird or the bird to the environment? In "The Laying Hen and Its Environment" (Ed. R. Moss). (Martinus Nijhoff, The Hague). pp. 19–42.

Freeman, B.M. and Manning, A.C.C. 1979. Stressor effects of handling on the immature fowl. Res. Vet. Sci., 26, 223-226.

Gallup, G.G. 1977. Tonic immobility: the role of fear and predation. Psychol. Rec., 27, 41-61.

Gallup, G.G., Cummings, W.H. and Nash, R.F. 1972. The experimenter as an independent variable in studies of animal hypnosis in chickens (Gallus gallus). Anim. Behav., 20, 166-169.

Gallup, G.G. and Suarez, S.D. 1980. An ethological analysis of open-field behaviour in chickens. Anim. Behav., 28, 368-378.

Gerrits, A.R., De Koning, K. and Migchels, A. 1985. Catching broilers. Misset Intern. Poult., 1, (5), 20-23.

Gray, J. 1971. The Psychology of Fear and Stress. (Weidenfeld and Nicolson, London).

Gross, W.B. and Siegel, P.B. 1979. Adaptation of chickens to their handler, and experimental results. Av. Dis.., 23, 708-714.

Hale, E.B. 1969. Domestication and the evolution of behaviour. In "The Behaviour of Domestic Animals" 2nd edition. (Ed. E.S.E. Hafez). (Bailliere, Tindall and Cassell, London). pp. 22-42.

Hemsworth, P.H. and Barnett, J.L. 1987. Human-animal interactions. In "Farm Animal Behavior" (Ed. E.O. Price). (Saunders, Philadelphia). pp. 339-356.

Hughes, B.O. and Black, A.J. 1976. The influence of handling on egg production, egg shell quality and avoidance behaviour of hens. Br. Poult. Sci., 17, 135-144.

Jones, R.B. 1987. Open field behaviour in domestic chicks (Gallus domesticus): the influence of the experimenter. Biol. Behav., 12, 100-115.

Jones, R.B., Duncan, I.J.H. and Hughes, B.O. 1981. The assessment of fear in domestic hens exposed to a looming human stimulus. Behav. Processes, 6, 121-133.

Jones, R.B. and Faure, J.M. 1981. The effects of regular handling on fear responses in the domestic chick. Behav. Processes, 6, 135-143.

Jones, R.B. and Hughes, B.O. 1981. Effects of regular handling on growth in male and female chicks of broiler and layer strains. Br. Poult. Sci., 22, 461-465.

McPherson, B.N., Gyles, N.R. and Kan, J. 1961. The effects of handling frequency on 8-week body weight, feed conversion and mortality. Poult. Sci., 40, 1526-1527.

Murphy, L.B. 1976. A Study of the Behavioural Expression of Fear and Exploration in two Stocks of Domestic Fowl. PhD Thesis, Edinburgh University, mimeographed.

Murphy, L.B. 1977. Responses of domestic fowl to novel food and objects. Appl. Anim. Ethol., 3, 335-349.

Murphy, L.B. and Duncan, I.J.H. 1977. Attempts to modify the responses of domestic fowl towards human beings. I. The association of human contact with a food reward. Appl. Anim. Ethol., 3, 321-334.

Murphy, L.B. and Duncan, I.J.H. 1978. Attempts to modify the responses of domestic fowl towards human beings. II. The effect of early experience. Appl. Anim. Ethol., 4, 5-12.

Murphy, L.B. and Wood-Gush, D.G.M. 1978. The interpretation of the behaviour of fowl in strange environments. Biol. Behav., 3, 39-61.

Reichman, K.G., Barram, K.M., Brock, I.J. and Standfast, N.F. 1978. Effects of regular handling and blood sampling by wing vein puncture on the performance of broilers and pullets. Br. Poult. Sci., 19, 97-99.

Ruegamer, W.R., Bernstein, L. and Benjamin, J.D. 1954. Growth, food utilization, and thyroid activity in the albino rat as a function of extra handling. Science, $\underline{120}$, 184–185.

Suarez, S.D. and Gallup, G.G. 1982. Open-field behavior in chickens. The experimenter is a predator. J. comp. physiol. Psychol., $\underline{96}$, 432–439.

Thompson, C.I. 1976. Growth in the Hubbard broiler: increased size following early handling. Devl Psychobiol., $\underline{9}$, 459–464.

Weininger, O. 1956. The effects of early experience on behaviour and growth characteristics. J. comp. physiol. Psychol., $\underline{49}$, 1–9.

Wolpe, J. 1958. Psychotherapy by Reciprocal Inhibition. (Stanford University Press, Stanford).

Wood–Gush, D.G.M. 1959. A history of the domestic chicken from antiquity to the 19th century. Poult. Sci., $\underline{38}$, 321–326.

Wood–Gush, D.G.M., Duncan, I.J.H. and Fraser, D. 1975. Social stress and welfare problems in agricultural animals. In "The Behaviour of Domestic Animals" 3rd edition. (Ed. E.S.E. Hafez). (Bailliere Tindall, London). pp. 182–200.

SESSION III : COGNITIVE ASPECTS

# SOCIAL RECOGNITION, SOCIAL DOMINANCE AND
# THE MOTIVATION OF FIGHTING BY PIGS

J. Rushen

Institut für Tierzucht und Tierverhalten
Trenthorst, 2061 Westerau,
Bundesrepublik Deutschland

## ABSTRACT

There is much evidence that a variety of animals can judge the relative fighting ability of an opponent on the basis of certain morphological cues such as comb size in domestic fowl. In initial fights, young pigs seem unable to make such judgements. However, they appear to be able to judge the relative fighting ability of an opponent from events that occur during a fight, in particular, the success each pig has in moving into a position for optimally delivering bites. The reduction in fighting that occurs as pigs become familiar occurs because the pigs accumulate information about relative fighting ability by remembering the outcome of earlier fights. Thus, the initial fighting between unacquainted animals is motivated by uncertainty about relative fighting abilities and can be considered a form of social exploration.

## INTRODUCTION

One source of social stress is the fighting that occurs when unacquainted animals are first brought together. Although this overt aggression is by no means the only, nor probably the most important, social source of stress, it can have a variety of undesirable consequences (reviewed by Fraser and Rushen, 1987; Petherick and Blackshaw, 1987). Most attempts to reduce this fighting have been purely "empirical" in that they have little theoretical justification, and, in general, they have not been hugely successful (Fraser and Rushen, 1987). I suggest that much of the problem lies in our lack of understanding of the fundamental motivation behind this fighting. In this paper, I discuss one source of ideas for increasing our understanding: theoretical studies of the evolution of "restrained" aggression.

ASSESSMENT OF FIGHTING ABILITY

Recent thinking on how aggressive behaviour has evolved has been stimulated by a series of mathematical models based on a cost/benefit analysis. These models have been used to explain how restrained or inhibited fighting, in which the animals refrain from fighting with maximum intensity, can evolve through benefits accruing to individual animals rather than through group or species selection. One idea that is central to many of these models is that animals will avoid fighting unless they have an acceptably high chance of winning. Consequently, animals should evolve means of judging their opponents' relative fighting ability ("resource holding potential" is the jargon). This is an old idea (e.g. Ewer, 1968) but recently the conditions under which it could evolve from natural selection have been formulated more precisely (e.g. Parker, 1974; Maynard Smith and Parker, 1976; Popp and De Vore, 1979; Enquist and Leimar, 1983).

Most of the interest has been on the ability of animals to make accurate judgements of relative fighting ability before a fight so that overt fighting can be avoided altogether. In general, it seems that many animals can make such judgements, using relative body size or some other anatomical cue to fighting ability such as horn or antler size, or through behavioural displays, pushing contests etc. Clutton-Brock and Albon (1979) and Davis and Halliday (1978) are two classic demonstrations of this ability. I have reviewed some of the evidence that domestic fowl can also make such judgements, possibly by estimating the size of an opponent's comb (Rushen, 1985).

Five lines of evidence show that such "perceptual" assessment occurs.

1). Animals should be able to settle disputes without fighting i.e. one animal should withdraw or submit immediately.

2). Such perceptual assessment should be less successful, that is fights should be more likely to occur, when animals are of similar fighting ability. As one example, Geist (1971)

showed that fights were more likely to occur between Mountain
Sheep that had similar sized horns.

    3). The animal with the highest  chance of winning (e.g.
the largest) should be more likely to start the fight.

    4). The anatomical cues or the behavioural displays used
by an animal to judge an opponent's fighting ability should
accurately predict actual fighting ability. For example, the
size of the comb of the domestic fowl may reflect levels of
testosterone production since injections, and external
applications of testosterone lead to growth of the comb.
Level of testosterone production seems to be one determinant
of fighting ability since injections of testosterone increase
fighting ability (Allee et al., 1939, 1955; Guhl, 1968) and
the social rank of  cockerels increases when sexual maturity
occurs (Rushen, 1982).

    5). Experimental changes to the cues should result in
predictable changes in the nature of the fights. Hens that
have had their combs removed tend to be defeated by hens with
intact combs (Marks et al., 1960), while birds with
artificially extended combs sometimes experience an increase
in their ability to win fights (Guhl and Ortman, 1953). Since
these changes should not have directly affected the fighting
ability of the birds, the results suggest that the changes
altered the "assessment" of strength made by their opponents.

    These five lines of evidence indicate such "perceptual
assessment" only when the observations are of the first
encounter between the animals. In interactions between
already acquainted animals, the evidence could instead be for
individual recognition. Indeed, the usual interpretation of
the effect of changing the comb is that these results show
that the comb is used to recognize individuals. This
interpretation is based, in part, on the mistaken belief that
the existence of stable dominance relationships must,
logically, be evidence for individual recognition. Barnard
and Burke (1979) and Wood-Gush (1987) criticize this
assumption. The problem of what is involved in "individual

recognition" is a difficult one (Alberts, 1985), and the
detailed empirical work that is needed to determine if a cue,
such as comb size, is a "status symbol", that is a cue about
relative fighting ability, or a cue used to discriminate
between individuals rarely has been done. The work of
Whitfield (1988) is an example of what is needed.

## ASSESSMENT OF FIGHTING ABILITY BY YOUNG PIGS

Recently, I did some experiments to look for evidence of
such assessment before a fight by young pigs. The results
were largely negative (Rushen, 1988). Pigs that differed
markedly in body weight were just as likely to fight as were
pigs of similar body weights. Furthermore, the pig that
eventually lost the fight was as likely to start the fight as
the eventual winner. This was unaffected by the size of the
weight difference between the two pigs. Since mammals may
require considerable learning and experience to develop the
complex skills needed to judge relative fighting ability
(Bekoff and Byers, 1985), the young age of the pigs may be
relevant.

However, there was evidence that the pigs were judging
their opponents fighting abilities during the fight. In such
cases, one animal would be expected to give up fighting
sooner where there was a large difference in fighting ability
between the two opponents. This was so for young pigs: the
eventual losers gave up fighting sooner when there was a
large weight difference between the two pigs (Rushen, 1988).
Furthermore, where assessment is occurring during a fight, it
should be possible to identify the particular behavioural
events that inform the combatants about their relative
fighting abilities (Enquist and Leimar, 1983; Enquist and
Jakobsson, 1986). That is, there should be some behavioural
difference between the ultimate winners and losers which is
apparent before the fight ends, and which should be larger
where the differences in fighting abilities between the two
combatants is larger. In fights between young pigs, the

number of bites received, and the success that each pig has in adopting offensive attacking positions (Rushen and Pajor, 1987), are the most likely candidates (Rushen, 1988).

## ASSESSMENT AFTER A FIGHT: WHY DO ANIMALS STOP FIGHTING?

Many have realized that an animal could use the outcomes of earlier fights with an opponent to judge relative fighting ability. This is important for the motivation of aggressive behaviour since the accumulation of information about relative fighting ability could explain why animals stop fighting as they become acquainted.

A common, alternative explanation is that animals stop fighting because they are no longer strangers. Archer (1976) has provided a stimulating model of how both fear and aggression are evoked in an animal by a discrepancy between what an animal expects to perceive in its environment and what it actually perceives. Initially, an encounter with a stranger results in such a discrepancy; increasing exposure to the stranger makes it more familiar, the discrepancy is reduced, and aggression is no longer evoked. This familiarity could be achieved through passive exposure; actual fighting need not occur. Zayan et al. (1983) have recently shown that domestic fowl from neighbouring cages show a reduced tendency to fight when they are brought together. Presumably, this occurs through habituation as the cage walls did not allow fighting to occur.

In some recent experiments, I explored whether the reduction in aggression that occurs as pigs become acquainted occurs through habituation or because the pigs are acquiring information about relative fighting ability (Rushen, 1988). For each pair of pigs, I observed two "paired-contests" separated by 24 h and looked, in detail, at the differences between the first and second encounters. The second time the pigs met fights were less likely to occur and, when they did, they were much briefer. This did not result from habituation or passive exposure: keeping the pigs in neighbouring pens so that they were in visual, auditory and olfactory contact (but could not fight) for 72 h or 14 d had little effect on the amount of fighting that occurred when the pigs were finally allowed to interact (c.f. Fraser, 1974). The fights were shorter the second time mainly because the loser stopped showing offensive behaviour earlier (see also Rushen, 1987). However, this was not because the winner was fighting more vigorously. Rather, the change in the behaviour of the loser seemed to result from the outcome of the first fight. On the first encounter, the eventual loser was just as likely to start the fight as the eventual winner. On the second encounter, the pig that had lost the first fight was now much less likely to initiate a second fight.

From this, I argue that the reduction in fighting that occurs as pigs become acquainted occurs because one pig has acquired sufficient information from previous fights to realize that it is of lower fighting ability than its opponent. Consequently this pig does not initiate aggression nor does it respond to aggression with counter aggression. Uncertainty about relative fighting ability is one of the causes of the aggression between unacquainted animals. This initial fighting can be considered as a form of social exploration, enabling the animals to learn some of the characteristics of their social companions.

CHANGE IN ASSESSMENT OR "LEARNING"

Talk of updating assessment of fighting ability as a result of repeated encounters may seem little more than restating, in more complicated jargon, the old and generally accepted idea that a defeated animal will learn from the outcome of a fight with that opponent and therefore be less likely to fight with that opponent in the future. Are there any advantages in talking of assessment? I believe there are several. First, it provides a conceptual link with assessment that may occur in initial encounters before learning has occurred. In this way, "assessment" is a more general concept.

Second, it raises the possibility of evolutionary pressures for using particular cues (i.e. those that accurately predict fighting ability) in learning to discriminate between individuals (Barnard and Burke, 1979; Caryl, 1982). This may explain why the comb of the chicken is used to discriminate between individuals (Candland, 1969; Guhl and Ortman, 1953). Third, the concept of assessment implies that animals seek to make the most accurate judgement of relative fighting ability.

It is quite common that the winner of a fight is not necessarily the strongest or most skillful; accidental and extraneous factors, such as the "peck-lag" effect (McBride, 1958), can be influential. Consequently, an animal wanting to make the most accurate judgement of fighting ability should not rely solely on the outcome of the first fight. The initial fights should play a limited role rather than a determining role in forming dominance relationships and the animal should seek to integrate information from a variety of sources (Barnard and Burke, 1979).

## ACKNOWLEDGEMENTS

I wrote this paper while I had an Alexander von Humboldt Fellowship. I thank Dr. Ladewig and Dr. Schlichting, and Prof. Dr. Dr. Smidt for providing me with facilities at Trenthorst.

## REFERENCES

Alberts, J. R. 1985. Ontogeny of social recognition: An essay on mechanism and metaphor in behavioral development. In "The Comparative Development of Adaptive Skills". (Ed. E. S. Gollin). (Lawrence Erlbaum, Hillsdale N. J.) pp. 95-135.

Allee, W. C., Collias, N. E. and Lutherman, C. Z. 1939. Modification of the social order in flocks of hens by the injection of testosterone propionate. Physiol. Zool., 14, 412-440.

Allee, W. C., Foreman, D., Banks, E. M. and Holabird, C. H. 1955. Effects of an androgen on dominance and subordinance in six common breeds of Gallus gallus. Physiol. Zool., 28, 89-115.

Archer, J. 1976. The organization of aggression and fear in vertebrates. In "Perspectives in Ethology vol. 3". (Eds. P. P. G. Bateson, P. H. Klopfer). (Plenum Press, New York). pp. 231-298.

Barnard, C. J. and Burke, T. 1979. Dominance hierarchies and the evolution of 'Individual Recognition'. J. theor. Biol., 81, 65-73.

Bekoff, M. and Byers, J. A. 1985. The development of behavior from evolutionary and ecological perspectives in mammals and birds. In "Evolutionary Biology vol. 19" (Eds. M. K. Hecht, B. Wallace and G. T. Prance). (Plenum Press, New York). pp. 215-286.

Candland, D. K. 1969. Discriminability of facial regions used by the domestic chicken in maintaining the social dominance order. J. comp. physiol. Psychol., 69, 281-285.

Caryl, P. G. 1982. Telling the truth about intentions. J. theor. Biol., 97, 679-689.

Clutton-Brock, T. H. and Albon, S. D. 1979. The roaring of red deer and the evolution of honest advertisement. Behaviour, 69, 145-170.

Davies, N. B. and Halliday, T. R. 1978. Deep croaks and fighting assessment in toads. Nature, 274, 683-685.

Enquist, M. and Jakobsson, S. 1986. Decision making and assessment in the fighting behavior of Nannacara anomala (Cichlidae, Pisces). Ethology, 72, 143-153.

Enquist, M. and Leimar, O. 1983. Evolution of fighting behaviour: decision rules and assessment of relative strength. J. theor. Biol., 102, 387-410.

Ewer, R. F. 1968. "Ethology of Mammals". Elek. Science, London.

Fraser, D. 1974. The behaviour of growing pigs during experimental social encounters. J. agric. Sci., Camb., 82, 147-163.

Fraser, D. and Rushen, J. 1987. Aggressive behavior. In "Farm Animal Behavior" (Ed. E. O. Price). (W. B. Saunders, Veterinary Clinics of North America: Food Animal Practice, Philadelphia). pp. 285-305.

Geist, V. 1971. "Mountain Sheep". (Chicago Uni. Press, Chicago)

Guhl, A. M. 1968. Social inertia and social stability in chickens. Anim. Behav., 16, 219-232.

Guhl, A. M. and Ortman, L. L. 1953. Visual patterns in the recognition of individuals among chickens. Condor, 55, 287-298.

Marks, H. L., Siegel, P. B. and Kramer, C. Y. 1960. Effect of comb and wattle removal on the social organization of mixed flocks of chickens. Anim. Behav., 8, 192-196.

Maynard Smith, J. and Parker, G. A. 1976. The logic of asymmetric contests. Anim. Behav., 24, 159-176.

McBride, G. 1958. The measurement of aggressiveness in the domestic hen. Anim. Behav., 6, 87-91.

Parker, G. A. 1974. Assessment strategy and the evolution of
    fighting behaviour. J. theor. Biol., 47, 223-243.
Petherick, J. C. and Blackshaw, J. K. 1987. A review of the
    factors influencing the aggressive and agonistic
    behaviour of the domestic pig. Aust. J. exp. Agric., 27,
    605-611.
Popp, J. L. and DeVore, I. 1979. Aggressive competition and
    social dominance theory: synopsis. In "The Great Apes"
    (Eds. D. A. Hamburg and E. R. McCown). (Benjamin/
    Cummings,California). pp. 317-338.
Rushen, J. 1982. The peck orders of chickens: How do they
    develop and why are they linear? Anim. Behav., 30, 1129-
    1137.
Rushen. J. 1985. Explaining peck order in domestic chickens.
    Bird Behav., 6, 1-9.
Rushen, J. 1987. A difference in weight reduces fighting when
    unacquainted newly weaned pigs first meet. Can. J. Anim.
    Sci., 67, 951-960.
Rushen, J. 1988. Assessment of fighting ability or simple
    habituation: what causes young pigs (Sus scrofa) to stop
    fighting. Aggr. Behav., in press.
Rushen, J. and Pajor, E. 1987. Offence and defence in fights
    between young pigs (Sus scrofa). Aggr. Behav., 13, 329-
    346.
Whitfield, D. P. 1988. The social significance of plumage
    variability in wintering turnstone Arenaria interpres.
    Anim. Behav., 36, 408-415.
Wood-Gush, D. G. M. 1987. Awareness and self-awareness in the
    domestic fowl and their relationship to animal welfare.
    In "Cognitive Aspects of Social Behaviour in the
    Domestic Fowl" (Eds. R. Zayan and I. J. H. Duncan).
    (Elsevier, Amsterdam). pp. 34-39.
Zayan, R., Doyen, J. and Duncan, I. J. H. 1983. Social and
    space requirements for hens in battery cages. In "Farm
    Animal Housing and Welfare". (Eds. S. H. Baxter, M. R.
    Baxter, J. A. C. MacCormack). (Martinus Nijhoff, The
    Hague). pp. 67-90.

# NEURAL PROCESSING OF VISUAL RECOGNITION OF INDIVIDUALS IN SHEEP

K. M. Kendrick

Agricultural and Food Research Council
Institute of Animal Physiology and Genetics Research
Cambridge Research Station
Babraham, Cambridge CB2 4AT, U.K.

ABSTRACT

The responses of single neurones in the temporal cortex of the brain of the conscious sheep to visual images of animals and humans have been studied using electrophysiological recording techniques. Results show that a small population of cells respond specifically to faces of animals and humans and that different cells discriminate between: (1) whether the faces shown have horns, and how large the horns are; (2) if the face shown is that of a sheep of the same breed and whether it is familiar and (3) if the face is that of a human or a dog. A further population of cells in this brain region responds to the sight of a human shape, rather than to the face. These latter cells are not simply specialised for visual recognition of humans, but are additionally responsive to the actions displayed by them. Thus the majority of cells only respond when a human approaches whereas relatively few do so when it remains stationary or withdraws. These results not only provide important insights into the neural processing of visual recognition in animals but also clearly illustrate the effects of social learning on optimising the way socially relevant distinguishing features (such as horns), and actions (approach/withdraw) are specifically coded for, at a sensory level, so that appropriate behavioural or emotional responses can be made with the minimum delay.

INTRODUCTION

While visual recognition of individuals is a well accepted fact in human and non-human primates less importance has been given to this form of recognition in non-primate mammals where considerably more emphasis has been placed on audition and olfaction. Clearly it would be wrong to suggest that auditory and olfactory mechanisms for individual recognition are unimportant in many of these species, but it would be equally wrong to ignore the visual system in this respect. Sheep, in common with many other domestic animals, have excellent visual acuity and probably even good colour vision and are therefore perfectly equipped to distinguish individuals using this sense. In sheep, the primary visual system in the brain is also fully developed and functional at birth (Ramachandran et al., 1977) and so it can be employed at the outset of post-natal life in the complex business of recognising, and making appropriate behavioural reactions to, other individuals and objects in their environment.

What evidence is there that sheep use their visual sense to aid in the recognition of objects and individuals? Firstly, it has been shown that sheep can perform complex discrimination learning tasks in the laboratory (Baldwin, 1981) and other electrophysiological experiments carried out in this laboratory have shown that cells in other areas of the brain, the lateral hypothalamus and zona incerta, respond differently to the sight of different foods (Kendrick and Baldwin, 1986). The most compelling evidence for the use of visual cues for individual recognition of other animals comes from ethological work in this laboratory showing that ewes primarily use visual cues from the head region to recognise their lambs. Thus, in experiments in which  different parts of the lamb´s body were systematically coloured black, it was found that the ewes only experienced difficulty in recognising their lambs when the whole body or just the head were coloured (Alexander and Shillito, 1977). Other evidence comes from studies showing that perception of the presence, and size, of horns gives information concerning dominance and gender in horned ungulates (Collias, 1956; Geist, 1968; Lincoln, 1972). Sheep are also known to form brief consortships with other sheep and have been shown to prefer to stay with members of their own breed (Shillito Walser et al., 1981; Winfield and Mullaney, 1973). It would seem probable that the processes of recognition necessary for identifying specific individuals would also partly involve the use of facial cues.

The temporal cortex of the brain has been identified, in sub-human primates and man, as an important region for the control of complex visual recognition. The temporal cortex receives projections from primary visual cortical areas and, in the monkey, a small population of cells in this region has been found to respond preferentially to the sight of monkey and human faces (Bruce et al., 1981; Gross et al., 1972; Perrett et al., 1982, 1987). Damage to this region in humans is often associated with problems in facial recognition (Meadows, 1974; Whiteley and Warrington, 1977). This type of high level cognitive processing of visual images was previously thought to be unique to primates. However, given the behavioural evidence for the importance of the face for recognition in sheep, and the fact that this species also possesses a temporal cortex, even though less well developed than that of a primate, led us to carry out a series of electrophysiological recording experiments to investigate the types of responses shown by single cells in this brain region in the sheep. Some of the results of these studies have already been published (Kendrick and Baldwin, 1987).

MATERIALS AND METHODS

Six adult Dalesbred sheep were used in the study. These animals were surgically prepared for conscious single-unit recording, under general anaesthesia and with sterile precautions, as previously described (Kendrick and Baldwin, 1986,1987). Recordings were made with the animals conscious and comfortably suspended in a canvas hammock and head movement was prevented by anchoring the insensitive portion of the sheep´s horns to the frame of the hammock. Single-unit activity was then recorded from cells in the temporal cortex using tungsten microelectrodes insulated with glass.

Visual stimuli were presented to the animals by means of a slide projector with the use of a back-projection screen (0.6 m wide and 0.4 m high) placed with its centre at eye level, 1 m directly infront of the animal. A number of different facial images (see Fig. 2A) were then presented, each for 5 seconds, either stationary or slowly moving horizontally across the screen (0.2 Hz). In this way, the images were presented in the most accurate part of the sheep's visual field, involving the area centralis of both eyes. The animals were clearly able to focus on the images presented and a few of the animals even vocalised when they saw the faces of other sheep, particularly familiar individuals. A Prontor shutter placed between the projector and the screen allowed automatic stimulus presentation as well as the recording of the response latencies of cells to the pictures. For each cell, each stimulus was presented 2-3 times, and the firing rate for the 5 seconds immediately prior to stimulus presentation was compared to that during the 5 seconds when the stimulus was presented. A mean percentage change in firing rate was then calculated. Where cells were found not to respond to the sight of faces a second series of tests was carried out to ascertain if they would respond to the sight of a human figure which either moved towards or away from the sheep or, alternatively, remained stationary. The neuroanatomical placement of recording electrodes in the temporal cortex was confirmed histologically at the end of the experiments.

## Criteria for responses to faces or human shapes

A cell was defined as responding preferentially to faces if it did not also respond to other arousing stimuli (loud noise, puff of air in the face or food) or projected images of either stationary or moving visual stimuli such as checkerboards or line gratings. These cells were also required to be unresponsive to pictures of sheep that showed the animal's body but not the head. Cells which fulfilled the above criteria were then tested for their responses to each of the 14 faces shown in Fig. 1A. These included horned sheep (Mouflon, Barbary, Dalesbred and Welsh Mountain) and goats (Saanen), non-horned sheep (Clun Forest and Finnish Landrace), pigs, sheepdogs and humans. To test for the effects of familiarity animals were shown pictures of both familiar (the sheep housed in the pen directly opposite the experimental animal) and unfamiliar Dalesbred sheep. Faces were presented not only in the normal orientation but upside down as well. In all cases, stimuli were presented randomly at one minute intervals with the room darkened.

Cells that did not respond to faces were also tested for their response to the sight of a human figure which was either stationary or moving towards or away from the experimental animal. For a cell to be classified as responding specifically to the sight of a human shape it was required not to additionally respond to the sight of objects or food, other arousing stimuli (loud noises or puff of air in the face) or the approach of a human in the dark.

RESULTS

Out of a total of 610 cells recorded from the temporal cortex of 6 sheep, 42 responded preferentially to facial stimuli and a further 48 responded preferentially to the sight of the human shape. The neuroanatomical region where these cells were found is shown in Fig.1.

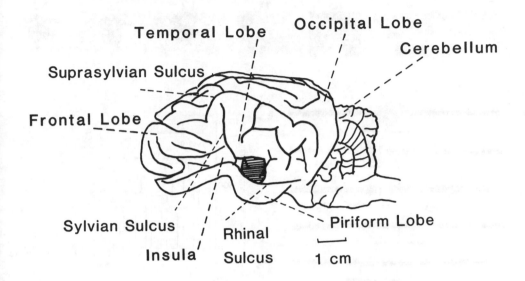

Fig. 1 Schematic drawing of a sagittal view of a sheep brain showing the location (shaded area) of cells in the temporal cortex responding to the sight of faces or the human shape. The area is just posterior to the sylvian sulcus and dorsal to the rhinal sulcus. (Adapted from Kendrick and Baldwin, 1987).

Neuronal responses to faces

Cells responsive to facial stimuli could be divided into four distinct types. The predominant type of response (21 cells) was for the cell to change its firing rate almost exclusively following presentation of pictures of horned animals (see Fig. 2C). Fig. 2B shows an example of the actual response profiles of one of these cells to each of the experimental stimuli. Both these figures clearly illustrate that only the horned animals are effective stimuli and that the animals with the largest horns (Mouflon and Barbary) are the most potent stimuli. An additional analysis was carried out on these cells using line drawings of a sheep with either large, medium sized or no horns (12,13 and 14 in Fig. 2A). Figs. 2B and C clearly show that the best response is evoked by the drawing with the large horns. These cells were not responding to the horns by themselves since they had to be presented in the context of an actual face in order to evoke a response. A second type of cell (8 cells) responded almost exclusively to

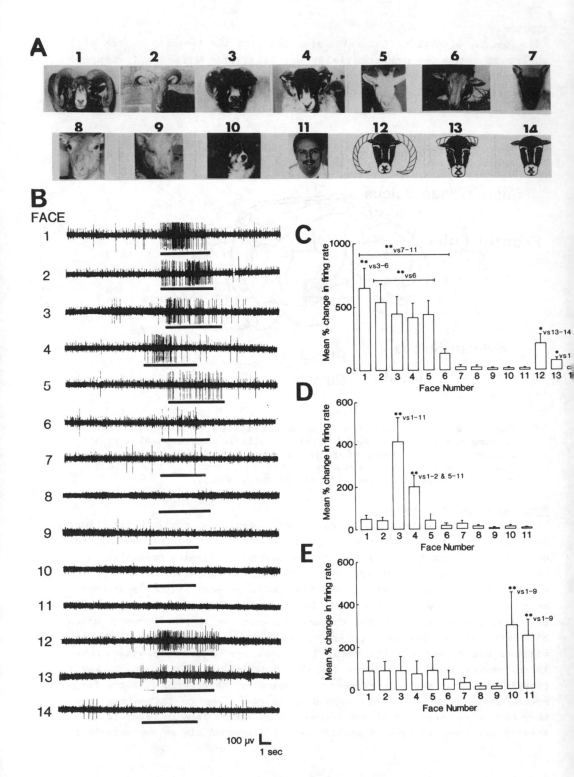

**A**

1 2 3 4 5 6 7

8 9 10 11 12 13 14

**B**

FACE

1

2

3

4

5

6

7

8

9

10

11

12

13

14

100 μv ⌐
1 sec

**C**

1000

**vs7-11

**vs3-6    **vs6

Mean % change in firing rate

0

1 2 3 4 5 6 7 8 9 10 11 12 13

Face Number

*vs13-14

*vs1

**D**

600

**vs1-11

**vs1-2 & 5-11

Mean % change in firing rate

400

200

0

1 2 3 4 5 6 7 8 9 10 11

Face Number

**E**

600

**vs1-9

**vs1-9

Mean % change in firing rate

400

200

0

1 2 3 4 5 6 7 8 9 10 11

Face Number

Fig. 2 (A) Facial stimuli used: 1. Mouflon, 2. Barbary, 3. Familiar Dalesbred, 4. Unfamiliar Dalesbred, 5. Saanen Goat, 6. Welsh Mountain, 8. Finnish Landrace, 9. Pig, 10. Sheepdog, 11. Human, 12-14 drawings of sheep with different sized horns. (B) Traces showing a single cell which responds best to the presentation of horned animals. Stimulus presentation is indicated by the black bar under each trace and the vertical deflections show action potentials produced by the cell. The numbered stimuli correspond to (A). (C) Histograms show mean (+ S.E.M.) percentage changes in the firing rates of 16 out of the 21 cells responding best to the faces of horned animals. Data for responses to the schematic drawings (11,12 and 13) are from 6 of these cells. (D) Same as (C), but for 8 cells responding best to the faces of Dalesbred sheep, particularly familiar ones. (E) Same as (C) but for 7 out of 9 cells responding best to the faces of humans and sheepdogs. Numbers under histograms identify the actual faces shown. Statistics: ** P < 0.01 and * P < 0.05 (Wilcoxon test) compared to the number of the facial stimulus indicated to the right of the asterisks. (Adapted from Kendrick and Baldwin, 1987).

the faces of Dalesbred sheep (i.e. the same breed as the experimental animal). In addition it was found that the familiar Dalesbred face was a more potent stimulus than the unfamiliar one (see Fig. 2D). Fig. 3 shows the responses of a single cell of this type which clearly increases its firing rate after the presentation of a familiar animal but does not respond to other horned animals. For 3 of the cells the effect of familiarity was confirmed using a further two sets of familiar/unfamiliar face pairings. A third type of cell (9 cells) responded most strongly to the sight of human and sheepdog faces (see Fig. 2E) and although there was additionally some tendency to respond to the presentation of the faces of horned animals this was not significant. A further analysis was carried out on two of these cells responding to human faces to investigate which components of the face were the most important for evoking the neuronal response. The responses of one of these cells to drawings of different components of the human face on a white card, are shown in Fig. 4. These data show that a correctly orientated outline of the face is the most important feature and probably the eyes are the second most important. Thus, a drawing showing only a correctly orientated outline and eyes is as effective a stimulus as a drawing containing all the facial features. The last type of cell (3 cells) did not show any clear discriminatory responses between the different facial stimuli, although faces were more effective stimuli than other objects. All four types of these cells showed considerable reductions in their responses to faces when they were presented upside down, providing further evidence for the specificity of their responses. All the faces presented in the study were shown frontally rather than in profile. However, in a few cases responses to profiles of faces were recorded although these were generally less intense than those shown to the frontal view of the same face. The latencies of the neuronal response to the visual presentation of the faces were extremely short,

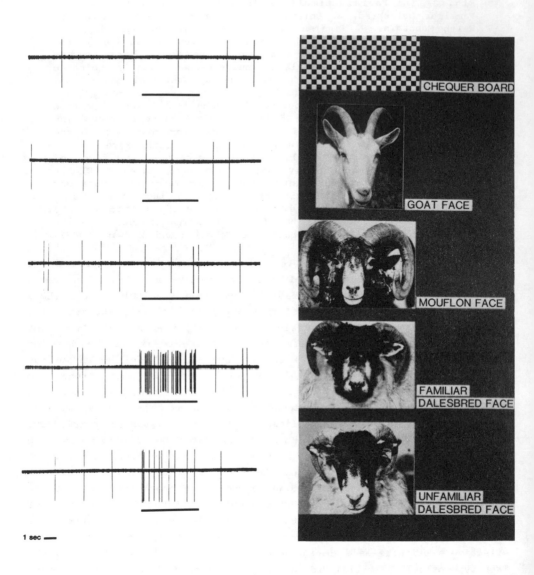

1 sec ▬

Fig. 3    Cell responding best to the sight of the faces of
Dalesbred sheep, and particularly those of familiar individuals.
The left side of the figure shows traces of a single cell´s
response to the facial, and control stimuli, shown on the right.
The horizontal bars under the traces show the period of stimulus
presentation and the vertical deflections the action potentials
produced by the cell.

ranging between 80 and 180 msec from the time that the images were first projected on the screen. The neuronal responses did not generally outlast the period of stimulus presentation (i.e. 5 seconds) but, with longer presentation periods, the response magnitude diminished.

## Neuronal responses to the human shape

Of the 45 cells found to respond specifically to the sight of the human shape, 29 required that the human was moving towards the animal in order for the stimulus to be effective and 8 only responded when the human moved away from the animal. Only 8 cells responded to the sight of a stationary human. All of these cells responded equally well to the human stimulus when the back view was presented instead of the front view, or when the head and shoulders were covered. Equally, these cells did not distinguish between different humans and did not respond to individual body parts presented in isolation (e.g. arms or legs). The one factor which was of importance was posture. Thus, there was a reduction, or abolition, of neuronal response when the human was seen in a quadrupedal posture as opposed to the normal bipedal one. Fig. 5 shows an example of a single cell which responds to an human approaching in the bipedal and not quadrupedal posture. In general these cells were not influenced by specific attributes of the human figure seen, however two cells showed a clear potentiation in their firing rate change when the individual seen was wearing a white laboratory coat (an item of clothing normally worn by experimenters and not by the people responsible for feeding and cleaning out the animals!).

## DISCUSSION

These results provide the first clear evidence that the temporal cortex of the sheep is involved in the processing of complex visual images associated with individual recognition. In this respect therefore this brain region would appear to play a similar role in sheep as it does in human and sub-human primates. The responses of these temporal cortical cells to faces and human shapes show remarkable similarities with those reported in monkeys (Bruce et al., 1981; Gross et al., 1972; Perrett et., 1982,1987). The visual features which trigger the cells to respond illustrate the important influence of social learning on the way the sheep's brain encodes this vital information. The first point to emphasise is that these cells respond extremely quickly to these visual stimuli (in < 180 msec) and they therefore provide the means to recognise an individual and show the appropriate behavioural or emotional reaction in the minimum possible time. However, not all individuals are equally important to respond to and therefore social learning biases the animal's response priorities in favour of individuals or objects that require the most immediate attention. Thus, the majority of cells which respond to the sight of faces are specialised for detecting the presence and size of horns. In horned ungulates the size of horns gives information both on dominance (the

152

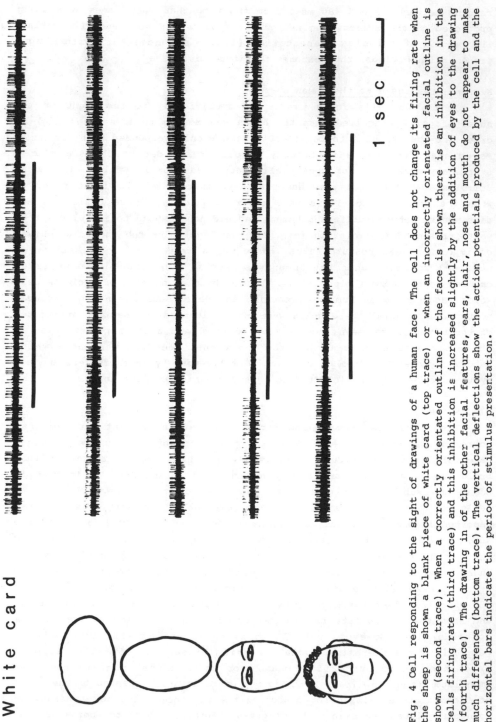

Fig. 4 Cell responding to the sight of drawings of a human face. The cell does not change its firing rate when the sheep is shown a blank piece of white card (top trace) or when an incorrectly orientated facial outline is shown (second trace). When a correctly orientated outline of the face is shown there is an inhibition in the cells firing rate (third trace) and this inhibition is increased slightly by the addition of eyes to the drawing (fourth trace). The drawing in of the other facial features, ears, hair, nose and mouth do not appear to make much difference (bottom trace). The vertical deflections show the action potentials produced by the cell and the horizontal bars indicate the period of stimulus presentation.

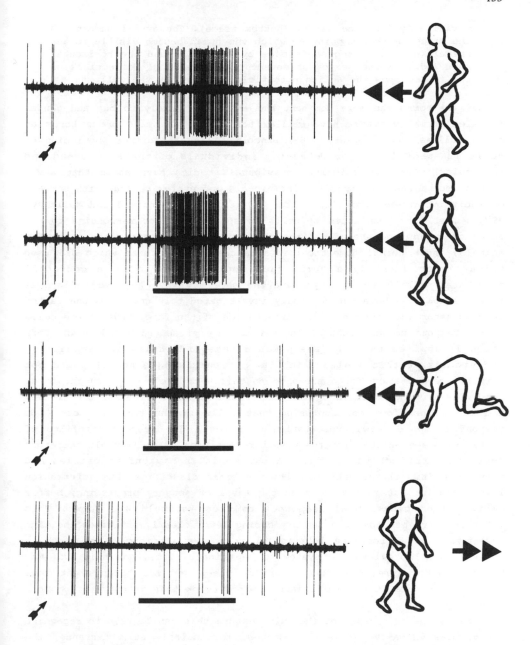

Fig. 5   Cell responding to the approach of a human figure. Traces on the left show that the cell responds to the approach of the human either forwards or backwards (top two traces) but not to a human approaching in a quadrupedal posture (third trace) or one

moving away from the animal (bottom trace). The arrows underneath the traces mark the point at which the human became visible to the animal (n.b. no response is made by the cell) and the horizontal bars indicate the period of movement. The vertical deflections on the traces show the action potentials produced by the cell.

larger the horns the more dominant the animal is likely to be) and gender (females normally either have smaller horns than the male or no horns at all - Collias, 1956; Geist, 1968; Lincoln, 1972). A further population of cells is specialised for detecting individuals of the same breed and particularly familiar animals. Behavioural studies have shown that sheep form consortships with specific individuals and prefer to stay with members of their own breed (Shillito Walser et al., 1981; Winfield and Mullaney, 1973). Lastly, a population of cells is specialised for responding to the faces of humans and sheepdogs, the two sources of potential threat to the animals, under normal domestic circumstances. The features which are used primarily to identify a human face would appear to be a correctly orientated profile and the eyes and the same may well be true for animal faces although we have not yet fully investigated this question. One factor that is important however is the orientation of the face. Thus, these cells do not respond to the sight of faces which are presented upside down. This strongly implies that the sheep would have difficulty in recognising individuals at this angle, which is not suprising since it would not normally be necessary for a sheep to do this. For the monkey, on the other hand viewing other animals upside down would be quite a normal occurrence, and it is therefore not suprising that cells in the temporal cortex do respond to upside down presentation of faces. The response profiles of these cells specialised for the visual recognition of individuals therefore accurately reflect the animal's known social behaviour priorities and provide additional insights into how the brain classifies this information into exclusive categories, even at the level of sensory processing, before emotional or behavioural responses to these stimuli are shown. This interpretative process at a sensory coding level clearly optimises the time taken to show appropriate behavioural responses (approach, avoid etc.), however, it also allows the system to be tricked. Thus, an individual may be wrongly interpreted as being another sheep and the sheep might move towards it before it had sufficient time to check this interpretation more carefully.

Faces are of course not the only feature that can be used to recognise individuals visually. In many instances, particularly at a distance, the face is not distinguishable or is actually turned away from view. How can visual recognition occur under these circumstances ? One answer to this question would appear to be through the perception of body shape and posture. As in the monkey (Perrett et al., 1985), the fact that a similar number of cells in the temporal cortex of the sheep respond to the sight of a human shape as do to faces illustrates the importance of this means of identification. These cells have clearly learned to respond to the human shape in such a way that they are capable of coping with a variety of different guises in which a human can appear (i.e. back view presented instead of front, head covered, different clothes, male or female etc.). The only way that they can be made to fail to make a response to the sight of a human is if the human radically changes his normal bipedal posture and goes on all fours. Sheep are not used to seeing humans adopt this posture and it is therefore not suprising that these cells fail to respond in these circumstances. With certain limitations therefore, it can be seen that these cells are specialised not for recognising particular individuals but a whole class of objects, namely humans. Obviously, the significance of the appearance of a human will vary, from a sheep´s point of view, depending upon what the human is doing. An approaching human is, for example, a much more important stimulus for a sheep than a stationary one or one moving away from it. It is therefore interesting to find that the majority of temporal cortex cells respond to an approaching human figure rather than a stationary or withdrawing one. These cells are therefore not merely specialised for aiding in the visual recognition of humans, but for recognising them in the context of the actions they are performing (i.e. approaching, withdrawing etc.). Once again therefore, visual stimuli are being coded in such a way that the appropriate behavioural response is triggered in the minimal possible time. We would expect to find similar cells which respond to the sight of sheep figures, however we have yet to test this hypothesis.

In summary therefore, the sheep possesses specialised neural circuitry for the recognition of individuals similar to that of sub-human primates, and probably man. The visual processing of these complex images is clearly influenced by learning, and there is a remarkable correlation between factors which have been shown by ethological studies to be important for the sheep and those which influence the response profiles of these cells. These types of study on the brain can therefore provide us with important insights into the ways that sheep, and other animals, view and interpret the world around them.

REFERENCES

Alexander, G. and Shillito Walser, E. 1977. Importance of visual cues from various body regions in maternal recognition of the young in Merino sheep (Ovis aries). Appl. Anim. Ethol., 3, 137-143.
Baldwin, B.A. 1981. Shape discrimination in sheep and calves. Anim. Behav., 29, 830-834.
Bruce, C.J., Desimone, R. and Gross, C.G. 1981. Visual properties of neurones in a polysensory area in the superior temporal sulcus of the macaque. J. Neurophysiol., 46, 369-384.
Collias, N.E. 1956. The analysis of socialization in sheep and goats. Ecology, 37, 228-239.
Geist, V. 1968. On the inter-relation of external appearances, social behaviour and social structures of mountain sheep. Zeit. Tier. Psychol., 25, 199-215.

156

Gross, C.G., Rocha-Miranda, C.E. and Bender, D.B. 1972. Visual properties of neurons in inferotemporal cortex of the macaque. J. Neurophysiol., 35, 96-111.

Kendrick, K.M. and Baldwin, B.A. 1986. The activity of neurones in the lateral hypothalamus and zona incerta of the sheep responding to the sight or approach of food is modified by learning and satiety and reflects food preference. Brain Res., 375, 320-328.

Kendrick, K.M. and Baldwin, B.A. 1987. Cells in temporal cortex of conscious sheep can respond preferentially to the sight of faces. Science, 236, 448-450.

Lincoln, G.A., 1972 The role of antlers in the behaviour of the Red deer. J. Exp. Zool., 182, 233-250.

Meadows, J.C. 1974. The anatomical basis of prosopagnosia. J. Neurol. Neurosurg. Psychiat., 37, 489-501.

Perrett, D.I. Mistlin, A.J. and Chitty, A.J. 1987. Visual neurones responsive to faces. Trends in Neurosci., 10, 358-364.

Perrett, D.I., Rolls, E.T. and Caan, W. 1982. Visual neurones responsive to faces in the monkey temporal cortex. Exp. Brain Res., 47, 329-342.

Perrett, D.I., Smith, P.A.J., Mistlin, A.J., Chitty, A.J., Head, A.S., Potter, D.D., Broennimann, R., Milner, A.D. and Jeeves, M.A. 1985. Visual analysis of body movements by neurones in the temporal cortex of the macaque monkey: a preliminary report. Behav. Brain Res., 16, 153-170.

Ramachandran, V.S., Clarke, P.G.H. and Whitteridge, D. 1977. Cells selective to binocular disparity in the cortex of newborn lambs. Nature, 268, 333-335.

Shillito Walser, E., Willadsen, S. and Hague, P. 1981. Pair association between lambs of different breeds born to Jacob and Dalesbred ewes after embryo transplantation. Appl. Anim. Ethol., 7 351-358.

Whiteley, A.M. and Warrington, E.K. 1977. Prosopagnosia: a clinical, psychological and anatomical study in three patients. J. Neurol. Neurosurg. Psychiat., 40, 394-430.

Winfield, C.G. and Mullaney, P.D. 1973. A note on the social behaviour of a flock of Merino and Wiltshire horn sheep. Anim. Prod., 17, 93-95.

THE EFFECT OF SOCIAL RECOGNITION UPON AGGRESSION
AND CORTICOSTEROID RESPONSES IN TRIADS OF PIGLETS

R. ZAYAN

Unité de Psychobiologie
1, Place Croix du Sud
B-1348 Louvain-La-Neuve (Belgium)

## ABSTRACT

The mixing of unfamiliar conspecifics is known to induce aggression, in particular figths, and to elevate levels of corticosteroid responses indicative of physiological stress. The present paper reports a series of experiments testing whether these behavioural and hormonal indicators of social stress would be specifically affected by social strangeness and familiarity. Accordingly, triads of weaned piglets were formed, in pens previously unknown to them, according to 3 conditions of grouping: - animals selected from the same litter (familiar individuals); - animals selected each from a different litter (unfamiliar individuals); - animals selected to form mixed triads, with two former littermates and one stranger taken from a different litter. In all triads, the animals were of same sex and strain, and of similar body weight and previous agonistic status. As a general rule, reciprocal aggression and plasma cortisol concentrations were significantly higher among the triads of strangers than among the mixed triads, and higher among the latter than among the triads of familiar animals. These results were interpreted in terms of social recognition, i.e. as the discrimination by a group member between a former littermate and an unfamiliar but equivalent conspecific. The results were also interpreted in terms of individual recognition in the triads of former littermates, where an animal discriminated between two familiar group-members as being particular conspecifics. It was concluded that social strangeness induced or facilitated social stress, whereas social familiarity inhibited aggressive interactions and reduced physiological stress; in other words, social recognition presumably operated to control social stress. So, regrouping former littermates for the start of the fattening period could act to alleviate social stress under husbandry conditions of overall environmental stress.

## INTRODUCTION

Social stress has been almost inevitably attributed to aggression,

particularly to fights, in the literature on farm animals (see, e.g. Fraser

and Rushen, 1987). And, agonistic interactions were most often reported to

157

be induced by artificial conditions of competition and by experimental disruption of social stability, e.g. by changing animals from one group to another, using a procedure that confounds two causes of social stress: that of associating unfamiliar conspecifics, but also that of transferring a strange intruder into the home area of a group of familiar residents not subjected to handling. Because aggressive interactions can cause physiological stress, the onset of fights is often considered to provide evidence (or, at least, reliable indication) of social stress. It is, however, admitted that social stress was not studied in pigs and in other farm animals as thoroughly as it was in poultry, and even more in laboratory rodents (Wood-Gush, 1983; Fraser and Rushen, 1987).

Crowding and social strangeness are often recognized as the main causes of social stress (Craig et al., 1969). The effects of density on aggression, hormonal responses and production indices of pigs were investigated in some detail (Bryant and Ewbank, 1972; Ewbank and Bryant, 1972; Warnier and Zayan, 1985, and references cited therein). More recently, the mixing of unacquainted pigs was chosen as an experimental paradigm suitable for studying social stress. Indeed, it consistently induces fights in adults as well as in piglets (Friend et al., 1983; Mc Glone, 1985; Rushen and Pajor, 1987), and it is followed by a significant increase in levels of plasma corticosteroids (Arnone and Dantzer, 1980; Blecha et al., 1985), by injuries, by reduced growth rate and by other detrimental effects (Mc Glone and Curtis, 1985; Mc Glone et al., 1986).

Grouping pigs of similar body weight selected from different litters is a common husbandry practice; such groups of unfamiliar conspecifics are formed, first when weaned piglets are to begin the fattening period, and subsequently when fattened pigs are to be taken to slaughter (Graves et al., 1978; Moss, 1978, 1980; Friend et al., 1983; Warris and Brown, 1985). One means of reducing aggression is to keep weaned piglets in intact litter groups as growing pigs or, at least, to form groups from a small number of litters (Friend et al., 1983). This procedure suggests that whereas social strangeness induces aggression and enhances stress, social familiarity would tend to reduce them, and in particular fights (Meese and Ewbank, 1973). Even when strangers are grouped, aggression strongly declines after the first day following the encounters (Graves et al., 1978; Meese and Ewbank, 1973; Mc Glone, 1986). A similar effect is found after a brief repeated exposure to initially unfamiliar conspecifics (Fraser, 1974; Friend et al., 1983; Rushen and Pajor, 1987; Rushen, in press). In contrast, a return of individuals to their former group after a long period of separation reactivates aggressive responses (Ewbank and Meese, 1971). Even a passive exposure to neighbours (for a period of 3 days) housed in pens providing sensory information but not allowing behavioural interactions and bodily contact reduces aggression (Fraser, 1974), although a reduction of fighting is more pronounced after the animals did engage in fights (Rushen, in press). This result suggests that the sensory cues involved in social and/or individual recognition (Ewbank et al., 1974, for sight; Meese and Baldwin, 1975, for olfaction) contribute to the reduction of aggressive interactions and also probably to the formation of stable dominance hierarchies (Ewbank and Meese, 1971; Meese and Ewbank, 1972 and 1973).

Although the fighting behavioural patterns of experimentally grouped pigs has been well described (Mc Bride et al., 1964; Fraser, 1974; particularly Mc Glone, 1985, Rushen and Pajor, 1987 and Fraser and Rushen, 1987), this suggestion that social strangeness induces aggression and enhances physiological stress was rarely tested. Zayan and Thinès (1984) compared the effects of mixing strangers to those of regrouping familiar pigs of same sex, age, weight and previous agonistic status. They found, both in pairs and in groups of 4 weaned piglets, that reciprocal aggression as well as plasma cortisol concentrations were very significantly increased among mixed strangers than among former littermates. Another result, from one of Rushen's (1987) experiments, confirms these findings for the case of fighting behaviour (no indices of physiological stress were recorded). Forming groups of 4 pigs by taking one large and one small piglets from each of two litters, and comparing the encounters between the large vs small unacquainted pairs to those of the large vs small pairs of littermates, Rushen found the mean duration of fighting to be about 4 to 7 times longer among the strange opponents. In all cases, the longest fights were recorded during the 1st hour following the groupings; after the 2nd hour, and, in the pairs of largest strangers after the 3rd hour, fighting was totally absent. Because, however, of the design that motivated this experiment, no data were available for the case of familiar group-members of symmetric body weights.

The present paper reports a series of experiments testing the hypothesis that social strangeness would induce or increase social stress (and not only aggressiveness, manifested by reciprocal aggression), whereas social familiarity would reduce social stress. Such facilitation and inhibition, respectively, of social stress would be the result of a control mechanism provided by an elementary cognitive process, namely social recognition, i.e. the discrimination by a piglet between a familiar and a strange conspecifics of symmetric properties. Triads of animals were formed, and it was also hypothesized that inhibition of aggression and alleviation of social stress would be most pronounced when individual recognition could operate among groups composed exclusively of former littermates. Social stress was investigated under the assumption that an increase of reciprocal aggression, expected among strangers, would be concomitant of an increase in plasma cortisol concentrations, traditionally regarded as a reliable indicator of physiological stress.

Rushen (1987) was mainly concerned by the effects of body weight asymmetries upon the frequency and duration of fighting behaviour among unfamiliar pigs. So, he was not specifically interested in forming samples of experimental pairs or groups composed exclusively of former littermates. Interestingly, Rushen's results with groups, composed of 2 familiar and of 2 unacquainted individuals, are somehow consistent with those of Zayan and Thines (1984) on tetrads of piglets of similar body weights. They recorded both unilateral and reciprocal aggression much more frequently among the members of the familiar tetrads than among the groups of 4 strangers. The plasma cortisol concentrations also tended to be more elevated among the members of the tetrads of unfamiliar pigs. Another result that bears out Rushen's is that both in the case of pairs and in the case of tetrads, more frequent aggression occurred among the strangers than among the former littermates immediately after the encounters were staged, and during the 4 subsequent hours fixed as period of observation for the experiments. A similar result was found by Rushen among his asymmetric dyads of familiar and of unfamiliar piglets forming his tetrads, the duration of mutual fighting being longer among the latter during the total 9hr period of observation, but this difference being most (about 5 times more) pronounced during the first 2 hours that followed the groupings. Rushen's results could be interpreted in terms of social discrimination among members of newly formed groups. It may have been the case that among the dyads of littermates, each animal recognized his familiar conspecific of asymmetric body weight from each of the asymmetric members of the other dyad. Such instance of social recognition could be quite accurate, as when the small (or the large) littermate distinguishes between his larger (or smaller) littermate and the large (or small) member of the other litter.

The experiments to be now reported could test for such an effet of social recognition among members of mixed triads, independently of an effect of body weight asymmetry. Triads either of familiar pigs or of strangers were also formed as controls.


## GENERAL OUTLINE OF THE EXPERIMENTS

A series of experiments was carried out during two years. Each time, between 6 and 9 litters of Pietrain piglets, reared by a local producer, were transported from their native pens to the pre-experimental pens of our piggery house, about one week after they had been weaned (in average, at the age of 34 weeks). The members of the original litters were kept together during their transport and were then introduced into the pre-experimental pens, where they remained as littermates for periods comprised between 7 and 12 days.

Animals of same sex, of very similar age, body weight, and of equivalent aggressive status (animals of intermediate ranks, the most aggressive and those manifesting most avoidance being excluded, were identified by observing agonistic interactions) were selected from litters of similar group-size to form triads in different pens. The experimental pens were unfamiliar to the animals, but they were located in the same room as the home pens and had the same structure and floor area (4 m²) as the latter. The animals were taken out of their home pens and guided, without receiving a tranquillizer, to the experimental pens located rather near (about 20 m) from their home pen.

During the whole period when the experiments were carried out, piglets were randomly assigned to 3 social conditions of testing: - as familiar individuals, selected from the same litters; - as strangers, selected each from a different litter; - as members of mixed triads, composed of two familiar individuals (littermates) and of a stranger. Half of the total number of triads formed according to these 3 experimental conditions served for the behavioural observations of agonistic interactions, conducted during either 3 hours or 4 hours following the formation of the groups. The other half of the formed triads served for the hormonal measures. In order to assay plasma cortisol concentrations, blood samples were collected 15-30 minutes after the groups were formed, 2 hours after the tests began, and 4 hours after the triads were formed; baseline control measures were collected from blood samples taken exactly 24 hours before the animals were tested. After the tests, all the animals were again placed in their initial home pens with their littermates.

The statistical comparisons were not made between all the members belonging to the 3 samples of triads, but between the members of each triad whose results corresponded to the median value of the three animals. It was, indeed, very likely that both the adrenocortical responses and the behavioural responses of each member of a triad statistically depended upon the respective responses of the two other group-members. Strictly speaking, only results obtained for triads, rather than for the individuals forming all the triads, could be considered representative of the 3 independent samples of experimental groups.

## GENERAL RESULTS

## COMPARISON BETWEEN FAMILIAR TRIADS AND MIXED TRIADS

The first series of experiments compared the effects of grouping three familiar individuals, selected from the same litters (E triads), to those of grouping two littermates (familiar animals $e^1$ and $e^2$) and one animal selected from a different litter (the strange individual c). These mixed groups will be referred to as the C triads on some tables and figures, whereas they will be referred to as the E + C triads on some other tables and figures, as indicated on the legends. The members of all formed triads were left together for a period of 3 hours following the groupings. Different samples of the two types of triads were formed for the observations of aggressive behaviour and for the tests to provide the hormonal measures of stress.

## Behavioural observations

The behavioural data, recorded on 14 E triads and on 14 C triads, are presented on Table 1 (median values). They show that mutual aggression (fights and/or reciprocal hits with flank or snout) were totally absent among familiar individuals, those of the E triads as well as the two ones in the C triads; the same result is found for the case of pushings (which was most often seen to occur as a mutual pattern). As to unilateral aggression (bites and/or hits causing flights in a group-member), it was never observed between the $e^1$ and $e^2$ piglets of the C triads, and it was occasionally observed, only during the 1st hour, among the members of the E triads. As a general rule, aggression was recorded between each of the $e^1$ and $e^2$ piglets and their strange group-member c (Table 1 naturally presents the median agonistic values calculated for the sample of all distinct familiar $e^1$ and $e^2$ individuals, whether or not they interacted with c). The median values of the C triads, obtained for the sums of the interactions recorded among all members of each triad, appear to be clearly higher than the corresponding medians of the E triads, particularly during the 1st and during the whole of the 3-hour period of observation. Table 2, which presents the statistical comparisons made between the two samples of triads (using the Fisher test: F, and the Mann-Whitney test : U, 1-tailed, applied to the total number of agonistic interactions recorded among all the triad members) strongly confirms this hypothesis. Table 2 does not mention the significantly higher ($p<0.001$) aggression which was manifested by the two familiar members of the C triads in comparison with the familiar members of the E triads. This result accounts for the difference found at the general level between the E and the C triads. Figure 1, which represents the direction of the agonistic interactions recorded during the 1st hour, illustrates the main results of the behavioural observations: - in the E triads, unilateral aggression was rarely observed (in only half of the groups), and reciprocal aggression (but not fights) occurred only in one group; - in the C triads, no aggression at all occurred between 9 dyads of familiar $e^1$ and $e^2$ animals, and reciprocal aggression (but not fights) occurred only in one group, whereas reciprocal aggression involving the strange c piglet was observed in all but one triad, and fights in 11 triads. These illustrations suggest an obvious result, namely that dominance-subordination relations, considered to have been established on the basis of significantly more frequent unilateral aggression and flight responses, should be more frequently inferred among the members of the C triads. Figure 2 shows that it was actually the case: agonistic dominance relations could be hypothesized in none of the 14 E triads, where it was found that unilateral aggression was either absent or too rare to allow a statistical comparison. In the 3 C triads where a similar result was found, it could also be attributed to many reciprocal interactions in which each animal initiated aggression about as frequently as its opponent, so that a statistical significant difference could not be found in this case either (the same occurred in many encounters between one of the familiar piglets $e^1$ or $e^2$ and the stranger c). In total, 16 dyadic dominance relations could be considered to have been established among the members of the C triads during the 1st hour that followed the groupings (against none among the dyads of the E triads).

From the behavioural observations it can be concluded that familiarity reduces aggression and flight responses among piglets reunited in a strange environment. Such inhibition of agonistic interactions was found among the former littermates of the E triads, but also among the two former littermates of the C triads. In contrast, each one of them tended to be involved in aggressive encounters with the strange conspecific which was placed with them in the same strange pens. Social strangeness, thus, very likely induces aggression, most often reciprocal (the piglet c also perceives $e^1$ and $e^2$ as strangers). As to social familiarity, its inhibitory effect on aggression could be ascribed to two perceptive processes. The simpler one is social recognition, by which in the C triads each one of the familiar animals $e^1$ and $e^2$ discriminates between its familiar conspecific and the strange conspecific c.    The more complex one    would be individual  recognition,   by

which in  the E  triads each  animal discriminates  between its  two familiar

group-members as being particular conspecifics,    each possessing an array of

individual properties.  That such process might have been operative among the

members of the E triads is suggested by  the data presented on Table 3,    and

specifically collected in the course of another experiment, where 12 familiar

triads were formed and observed during a period of 4 hours.   Despite the low

number of agonistic  interactions,  it was significantly found:   that these

were addressed by $e^1$ more to $e^2$ than to $e^3$,  and by $e^2$ more to $e^3$ than to $e^1$;

that these more often occurred between $e^1$ and $e^2$ than between $e^1$ and $e^3$,   and

also  more often  between  $e^2$ and  $e^3$  than  between $e^1$  and  $e^3$.  There  is,

therefore,  evidence that two members of the E triads ($e^1$,  $e^2$)  each treated

their other two partners as different individual conspecifics.

  The question  raised now is  whether social strangeness,   here associated

with  increased  aggressiveness  and/or   facilitated  aggression,   actually

corresponded to  (caused?)  stress,   whereas social  familiarity would  have

reduced  stress.  To  answer this  question,  an  indicator of  physiological

stress,   namely plasma  cortisol concentrations,   was  measured in  animals

forming rather  large samples  of triads  of the  same two  types.  The  most

relevant comparison in this respect was to be made between the members of the

familiar triads and the two familiar members of the mixed triads. Indeed, the

former very rarely engaged in agonistic interactions and never in fights.   In

contrast,  the latter did not initiate  aggression as long as themselves were

concerned,   but were  systematically  involved  in aggressive  interactions,

particularly reciprocal, with the stranger.  It could, then, be expected that

these behavioural differences between the two samples of familiar individuals would be reflected by differences in adrenocortical responses. If the familiar members of the mixed triads showed higher cortisol concentrations, it could be concluded that social recognition between these $e^1$ and $e^2$ piglets does not suffice to reduce overall social stress present when (caused by?) fighting with a stranger, even though it was shown that $e^1$ and $e^2$ cooperated in their aggression against c. In contrast, individual recognition (or, at least, social recognition) among the three familiar members of the E groups would clearly have reduced overall social stress while (because?) it also inhibited aggressive experiences.

FIGURE 1

E – TRIADS (Familiar Piglets)

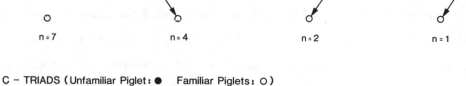

C – TRIADS (Unfamiliar Piglet: ● Familiar Piglets: ○)

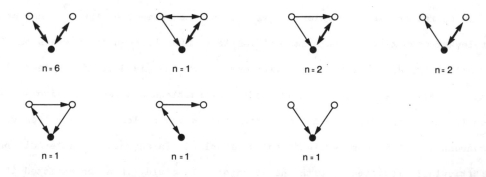

Agonistic interactions recorded 1 hour after piglets were grouped.

←→ Fights        Aggression: —→ unilateral        ←— reciprocal

FIGURE 2

Agonistic dominance relations established 1 hr after piglets were grouped
in strange pens.

Dominance (→) assessed from unilateral and more frequent aggression
(p < 0.05, binomial 2 - tailed test).

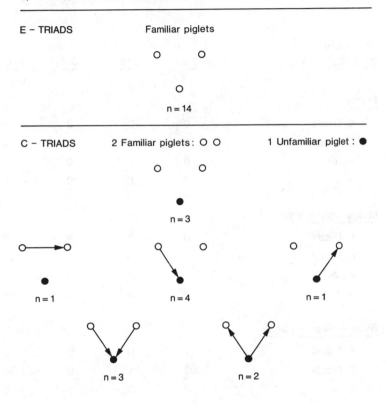

TABLE 1

Median values of behavioural patterns recorded in piglets grouped in triads as familiar individuals (E) or as 2 familiar individuals ($e_1$, $e_2$) associated with a stranger (c ; C triads).

| Hours after grouping : | 1st | 2nd | 3rd | 3 hours |
|---|---|---|---|---|
| **Fights** | | | | |
| E Triads | 0 | 0 | 0 | 0 |
| C Triads | 3 | 0 | 0 | 4 |
| $e_1$, $e_2$ | 0 | 0 | 0 | 0 |
| + c | 1 | 0 | 0 | 3 |
| **Mutual aggression** | | | | |
| E Triads | 0 | 0 | 0 | 0 |
| C Triads | 6 | 0 | 0 | 12 |
| $e_1$, $e_2$ | 0 | 0 | 0 | 0 |
| + c | 3 | 0 | 0 | 8 |
| **Bites + Hits → Flights** | | | | |
| E Triads | 1 | 0 | 0 | 2 |
| C Triads | 29 | 1 | 0 | 24 |
| $e_1$, $e_2$ | 0 | 0 | 0 | 0 |
| + c | 9 | 4 | 0 | 13 |
| **Pushings** | | | | |
| E Triads | 0 | 0 | 0 | 0 |
| C Triads | 1 | 0 | 0 | 3 |
| $e_1$, $e_2$ | 0 | 0 | 0 | 0 |
| + c | 0 | 0 | 0 | 0 |

TABLE 2

Statistical comparisons made between the behavioural patterns of piglets grouped as familiar individuals (E triads) or as 2 familiar individuals associated with a stranger (C triads). Significant differences express the tendency : C > E.

| E - C Comparisons | Period after grouping | | | |
|---|---|---|---|---|
| | | 1st Hour | | 3 hours |
| **Fights** | | | | |
| F | | p < 0.001 | | p < 0.001 |
| U : | 28 | p < 0.001 | 28 | p < 0.001 |
| **Mutual aggression** | | | | |
| F | | p < 0.001 | | p < 0.001 |
| U : | 11 | p < 0.001 | 11 | p < 0.001 |
| **Bites → Flights** | | | | |
| F | | p < 0.001 | | p < 0.001 |
| U : | 19 | p < 0.001 | 19 | p < 0.001 |
| **Hits → Flights** | | | | |
| F | | p = 0.005 | | p = 0.025 |
| U : | 0 | p < 0.001 | 3 | p < 0.001 |
| **Bites + Hits** | | | | |
| F | | p = 0.005 | | p = 0.025 |
| U : | 0 | p < 0.001 | 3 | p < 0.001 |
| **Pushings** | | | | |
| F | | p = 0.01 | | p = 0.025 |
| U : | 49 | p < 0.025 | 41 | p < 0.01 |

TABLE 3

E TRIADS : Familiar piglets $e_1$, $e_2$, $e_3$.
Frequency of agonistic interactions (hits/bites causing avoidance/flights) recorded during a 4 hr-period subsequent to the grouping of the members of same litters in strange pens.

| Pairs: | $e_1$-$e_2$ | | $e_1$-$e_3$ | | $e_2$-$e_3$ | |
|---|---|---|---|---|---|---|
| **Triad N°** | | | | | | |
| 1 | 1 — | 1 | — 1 | 1 | 1 — | 1 |
| 2 | 1 4 | 5 | — — | — | 5 — | 5 |
| 3 | 1 — | 1 | — — | — | 1 — | 1 |
| 4 | — 1 | 1 | — — | — | 1 — | 1 |
| 5 | — — | — | — — | — | 1 — | 1 |
| 6 | — 1 | 1 | — — | — | 1 — | 1 |
| 7 | 2 — | 2 | — — | — | 3 2 | 5 |
| 8 | — — | — | — — | — | — — | — |
| 9 | — — | — | — — | — | 2 — | 2 |
| 10 | 2 — | 2 | — — | — | 2 2 | 4 |
| 11 | 1 — | 1 | — 1 | 1 | 2 — | 2 |
| 12 | 2 — | 2 | — — | — | 1 — | 1 |

$$e_1 \rightarrow e_2 > e_1 \rightarrow e_3 \qquad p = 0.023$$
$$e_2 \rightarrow e_3 > e_2 \rightarrow e_1 \qquad p = 0.013$$
$$e_3 \rightarrow e_1 = e_3 \rightarrow e_2$$

$$e_1 - e_2 > e_1 - e_3 \qquad p = 0.023$$
$$e_2 - e_3 > e_1 - e_3 \qquad p < 0.008$$
$$e_1 - e_2 = e_2 - e_3$$

## Plasma cortisol concentrations

As can be seen from Table 4, the blood samples taken 24 hours before the groupings did not reveal any significant differences between the members of the familiar (E) triads and those of the mixed (here denoted E+C) triads. It can even be noted that the mean values fortuitously happened to be the same in the sample of 3 familiar piglets and in the sample of the two familiar members ($e^1$, $e^2$) of the mixed triads. But the blood samples taken subsequently revealed significant differences (using Mann-Whitney 1-tailed tests) between the piglets of the two types of triads. After 15 to 30 min following the groupings, plasma cortisol concentrations were lower among the familiar than among the mixed triads ($z=2.09$); they were, however, statistically equivalent (i.e. as high) in the strangers (c) and in the two familiar ($e^1$, $e^2$) members of these mixed E+C triads; logically, and most important, the mean levels of adrenocortical responses were significantly higher ($z=1.97$) among the two familiar $e^1$ and $e^2$ piglets exposed to the stranger c than among the three familiar piglets of the E triads. The same results were found 2 hours after the groups were formed ($z=2,33$; $z=1,97$ respectively). It may, therefore, be concluded that social familiarity cannot compensate for elevated social stress induced by the presence of a strange conspecific, and increased by aggressive interactions with such a stranger. Whether or not the two familiar conspecifics $e^1$ and $e^2$ did not themselves engage in aggressive interactions as a result of their mutual (social) recognition cannot be answered. What would seem to be more clearly established is that in the members of the familiar E triads, social recognition, and probably individual recognition, operates to reduce social stress by inhibiting mutual aggression (and vice-versa). Other experiments should test if such alleviation of social stress results from the absence of overt aggression, or more precisely from the presence of conspecifics readily recognized as familiar individuals. Similarly, control experiments should be carried out in order to test if the mere detection of a strange conspecific suffices to critically elevate corticosteroid responses in the two familiar members of the mixed triads, or if it is the aggression induced by the presence of a stranger that actually raises the level of hormonal responses indicative of stress. One cannot, in the context of the present experiments, assert that social stress was specifically induced by the perception of a strange conspecific, and was specifically reduced by the perception of a familiar conspecific (social recognition), or by the discrimination of two familiar conspecifics (individual recognition). It is, however, possible to conclude that the presence of strange (or of familiar) conspecifics, in conjunction with the reciprocal aggression that such presence induced (or inhibited), did very clearly increase (or decrease) plasma cortisol concentrations. These adrenocortical responses being classically considered as robust measures of physiological stress, the present experiments provided a specific paradigm for studies on social stress.

Before other experiments are summarized, it must be mentioned that the significant effect of grouping in the familiar and in the mixed triads was not found after 2 hours following the tests. After 4 hours, very similar plasma cortisol mean values were found in the familiar members of the E triads (35,4), in the familiar members ($e^1$, $e^2$) of the mixed triads (35,9), in the strangers (c) of the mixed triads (36,3), the mean values for all the members of these triads being slightly higher (36,1) than those of the members of the E triads. Another experiment was carried out with 14 familiar triads (E) and with 14 mixed triads (C). Half of the triads of each sample were tested for behavioural observations. Agonistic interactions were more frequently recorded among the members of the C triads during the 1st hour following the tests (fights: p=0.013; reciprocal aggression: p<0.001; bites: p=0.003; hits: p<0.001; bites+hits: p<0.001); after the 2nd hour following the tests, such result was found only for the total number of bites+hits: p=0.005; during the 3rd hour, more agonistic behaviour among the members of the C triads was still found, but less markedly and just for the case of hits (p=0.016). In the other half of the two samples of triads, in which plasma cortisol concentrations were assayed, the adrenocortical responses were found to be higher among all members of the C triads than in those of the E triads 30 min after the tests (mean values: 51,4 and 33,9; p=0.012) and 1hr30 min after the tests (mean values: 50,2 and 36,2; p=0.029), but not 2hrs30 min after the tests (mean values: 39,2 and 38,0). And, plasma cortisol levels appeared to be higher among the two familiar members of the mixed groups than among the members of the familiar E triads, 30 min after the tests (mean values: 49,6 and 33,9; p=0.05) but not later (1hr 30 min: 48,7 and 36,2; 2hrs 30 min: 39,0 and 38,0). Figure 3 represents the evolution of these differences. These results indicate that fluctuations of plasma cortisol concentrations reflecting concomitant changes in levels of agonistic responses may prove to be reliable indicators of social stress only during the period that immediately follows the association between familiar or strange conspecifics.

TABLE 4

Plasma cortisol concentrations (in ng/ml) of piglets tested in triads of familiar individuals (E), or in mixed triads (E + C) of 2 familiar ($e_1$, $e_2$) and 1 strange (c) individuals.

| Blood samples taken | E TRIADS N = 27 | | | E + C TRIADS N = 37 | | |
|---|---|---|---|---|---|---|
| | $e_1$ | $e_2$ | $e_3$ | $e_1$, $e_2$ | c | Triad |
| **Test - 24 hrs** | | | | | | |
| Means | | 32,9 | | 32,9 | 35,0 | 33,6 |
| **Test + 15-30 min** | | | | | | |
| Means | | 44,1 | | 54,9 | 54,7 | 54,8 |

Comparisons

| | E | $p = 0.024$ | $e_1$, $o_2$ |
|---|---|---|---|
| | E | $p = 0.018$ | E + C ($e_1$, $e_2$ = c) |

| **Test + 2 hrs** | | | | | | |
|---|---|---|---|---|---|---|
| Means | | 30,7 | | 38,5 | 40,1 | 39,0 |

Comparisons

| | E | $p = 0.024$ | $e_1$, $e_2$ |
|---|---|---|---|
| | E | $p = 0.010$ | E + C ($e_1$, $e_2$ = c) |

FIGURE 3

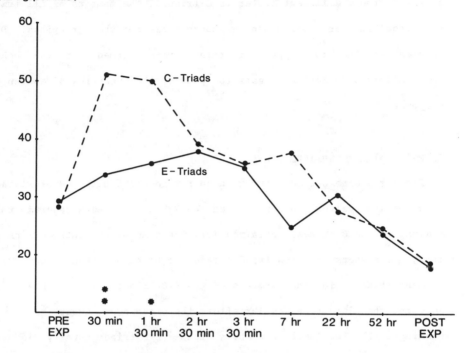

Plasma Cortisol concentrations
( in ng per mls )

Time after piglets were grouped in the E and C-Triads

E - Triads : 3 Familiar piglets
C - Triads : 2 Familiar piglets +1 strange piglet
Cortisol concentrations : C > E  ✸ p=0.01  ● p=0.03

COMPARISON BETWEEN TRIADS OF STRANGERS AND MIXED TRIADS

A second series of experiments compared the effects of grouping three strange individuals, selected from different litters (C triads), to those of grouping two familiar individuals ($e^1$, $e^2$) and one strange animal (c) selected from a different litter (E+C triads). The members of all triads were left together for a period of 4 hours following the groupings. Different samples of the two types of triads were formed for the behavioural observations and for the tests to provide the measures of adrenocortical responses.

Behavioural observations

The tests were carried out with 14 E triads and with 14 E+C triads. The data (median values) are presented on Table 5. As a general rule, the medians of the C triads, obtained for the sums of the interactions recorded among all members of each triad, tend to be higher than the corresponding medians obtained for the members of the E+C triads; this tendency is clear only for the data recorded 1hr after the groupings, except in the case of pushings. The two familiar members of the E+C triads usually did not engage in mutual aggressive interactions, and showed little bites and hits after 4 hrs. In contrast, each of these $e^1$ and $e^2$ piglets tended to interact aggressively with the stranger c.

The statistical comparisons, presented on Table 6, show that during the 1st hour that followed the test, the members of the two samples of triads did not differ in their rate of reciprocal aggression; only unilateral aggression (bites, bites+hits) was significantly higher among the members of the C triads than among those of the mixed triads (Mann-Whitney 1-tailed U tests).

This difference was not found for the whole of the 4-hour period of observation, whereas reciprocal aggression appeared then to have been higher among the triads of strangers (Fisher F as well as U tests, 1-tailed). Table 6 does not mention one result, namely that a strange piglet (c) engages in lesser aggressive interactions with two strange conspecifics familiar with each other ($e^1$, $e^2$) than does any of the strangers in the C triads with two other group-members also unknown to each other (p<0.01 in all cases where significant differences were found between the two samples of triads). This result is more informative than its corollary, namely that two familiar animals interact more aggressively with a stranger than do two strangers with a third, unfamiliar, group-member. But, the comparison between the mixed triads and the C triads does not provide results as specific as those arising from the comparison between the mixed triads and the E triads. The former lacks, by definition, an intermediate control condition in which mixed triads would be formed by grouping two strangers with one familiar animal. So, it is not possible to evaluate the behaviour (and hormonal responses) of unfamiliar individuals depending on whether they encounter a third strange conspecific or familiar animals; experiments with tetrads would be required for this purpose. Be that as it may, it can be globally concluded from the present comparisons that systematic strangeness among conspecifics increases aggression, and that partial familiarity significantly reduces it.

TABLE 5

Median values of behavioural patterns recorded in piglets grouped in triads of strange individuals (C) or as 2 familiar individuals ($e_1$, $e_2$) associated with a stranger (c ; E + C triads).

| Hours after grouping : | 1st | 2nd | 3rd | 4th | 4 hours |
|---|---|---|---|---|---|
| **Fights** | | | | | |
| E + C Triads | 4 | 0 | 0 | 0 | 4 |
| $e_1$-$e_2$ | 0 | 0 | 0 | 0 | 0 |
| + c | 1 | 0 | 0 | 0 | 1 |
| C Triads | 7 | 0 | 0 | 0 | 12 |
| **Mutual aggression** | | | | | |
| E + C Triads | 8 | 0 | 0 | 0 | 4 |
| $e_1$-$e_2$ | 0 | 0 | 0 | 0 | 0 |
| + c | 1 | 0 | 0 | 0 | 1 |
| C Triads | 10 | 2 | 0 | 0 | 15 |
| **Bites + Hits → Flights** | | | | | |
| E + C Triads | 21 | 11 | 8 | 3 | 58 |
| $e_1$-$e_2$ | 0 | 0 | 0 | 0 | 2 |
| + c | 18 | 3 | 1 | 2 | 27 |
| C Triads | 37 | 14 | 10 | 6 | 120 |
| **Pushings** | | | | | |
| E + C Triads | 1 | 0 | 0 | 0 | 2 |
| $e_1$-$e_2$ | 0 | 0 | 0 | 0 | 0 |
| + c | 0 | 0 | 0 | 0 | 1 |
| C Triads | 1 | 0 | 0 | 0 | 2 |

TABLE 6

Statistical comparisons made between behavioural patterns of piglets grouped as strange individuals (C Triads) or as 2 familiar individuals associated with a stranger (E + C triads). Significant differences express the tendency : C > E + C.

| | | Period after grouping | | | |
|---|---|---|---|---|---|
| E + C − C Comparisons | | 1st Hour | | 4 hours | |
| Fights | | | | | |
| | F | p > 0.05 | | | p = 0.05 |
| | U : | p > 0.05 | | 44 | p < 0.01 |
| Mutual aggression | | | | | |
| | F | p > 0.05 | | | p = 0.05 |
| | U : | p > 0.05 | | 44 | p < 0.01 |
| Bites → Flights | | | | | |
| | F | p > 0.05 | | | p > 0.05 |
| | U : | 53 | p < 0.025 | | p > 0.05 |
| Hits → Flights | | | | | |
| | F | p > 0.05 | | | p > 0.05 |
| | U : | p > 0.05 | | | p > 0.05 |
| Bites + Hits | | | | | |
| | F | p > 0.05 | | | p > 0.05 |
| | U : | 55 | p = 0.025 | | p > 0.05 |
| Pushings | | | | | |
| | F | p > 0.05 | | | p > 0.05 |
| | U : | p > 0.05 | | | p > 0.05 |

## Plasma cortisol concentrations

The medians and the mean values assessed in the piglets of the two samples of triads are presented on Table 7. As can be seen, the values of the two samples were equivalent 24 hours before the groupings were made. No significant differences were found 15 to 30 min after these tests began. However, significant differences which confirmed the behavioural results were found 2 hours after the triads were formed. Thus, adrenocortical responses were higher among the strange members of the C triads than among the familiar and strange members of the E+C triads. Besides, the strangers (c) of these mixed triads had lower plasma cortisol levels than those found in the strangers of the C triads. These findings suggest that social stress was increased among the members of triads composed of strangers only, whereas it was decreased in the mixed triads, as a result of the single strangers being engaged in lesser aggressive interactions with the two familiar members of these triads.

## EXPERIMENTS WITH ALL SAMPLES OF TRIADS TESTED SIMULTANEOUSLY. PLASMA CORTISOL CONCENTRATIONS

An experiment was designed to test the specific hypothesis that levels of adrenocortical responses would systematically increase as the number of unfamiliar piglets increased in a triad. Equivalently, it was hypothesized that social strangeness would correspond to (perhaps induce, or cause) higher indices of physiological stress. Knowing than these correspond to (perhaps are induced, or caused by) higher frequencies of aggression, it was hypothesized that increased social strangeness would actually correspond to increased social stress. Conversely, it was assumed that increased social familiarity would be reflected by reduced levels of adrenocortical response which, together with inhibition of aggressive responses, would provide a reliable indication that social stress was being alleviated. The medians and mean values of plasma cortisol concentrations assayed in the members of the 3 samples of triads are presented on Table 8. As can be seen, the concentrations obtained 24 hours before the animals were grouped did not markedly differ.

The statistical comparisons, shown on Table 9, reveal the following results. No significant differences were ever found between the familiar triads (E) and the mixed triads (E+C). This result totally contrasts with those found earlier, and shown on Table 4; whether 15-30 min or 2 hours after the groupings, the plasma cortisol levels are now equivalent in all members of the two samples of triads, as well as in the two familiar members of the mixed triads and in all three members of the E triads. It was, however, found as previously that the plasma cortisol levels were, in the mixed triads, equivalent in the two familiar animals ($e^1$, $e^2$) and in the stranger (c), which suggests that adrenocortical responses were increased in the two former littermates as a result of encountering a stranger. This suggestion would be supported if plasma cortisol concentrations were found to be significantly higher in the members of the triads of strangers (C) than in the members of the familiar triads (E); this was actually the case for the measures taken 2 hours following the tests. In addition to this novel finding, the abovementioned suggestion would be supported if plasma cortisol concentrations were found to be much higher in the members of the triads of strangers (C) than in the members of the mixed triads (E+C), because these included two familiar individuals. And, as was previously found (Table 7), this was actually the case 2 hours after the triads were formed (Table 9; see also Table 8: C=40,7 and 41,9; E+C= 32,3 and 31,7). The fact, however, that adrenocortical responses were also significantly higher among the strangers of the C triads than among the strange members (c) of the mixed triads after 2 hours (a result confirming the one previously found, and shown on Table 7) suggests that the presence of the two familiar animals in the mixed triads has reduced social stress in their strange (c) group-member. A look at Table 8 confirms this suggestion (c=35,8 and 32,5; C=40,7 and 41,9). Finally, a look at the median and mean values obtained 2 hours after the groupings indicates (Table 8) that the plasma cortisol concentrations tend to increase as the number of strange individuals in a triad increases (E triads = 30,5 and 29,8; E+C triads = 32,3 and 31,7; C triads = 40,7 and 41,9). The Kruskall-Wallis test, which was used (H= 9,82; $p<0.01$) prior to testing the differences between each of the 3 pairs of samples of triads (by means of 1-tailed U tests), could not properly test if such transitive trend was statistically significant. The Jonckheere-Terpstra test for ordered alternatives, specifically designed to test such a transitive trend, actually confirmed it very significantly (z= 2,65; p=0.004, 1-tailed).

Finally, it must be mentioned that behavioural observations were also carried out simultaneously in other piglets belonging to the 3 samples of triads E, E+C, and C (n=11 triads in each sample, observed during 4 hours). As could be predicted, the frequencies of fights, of reciprocal aggression and of unilateral agonistic interactions all followed a transitive trend, being significantly higher among strangers than among members of mixed groups and than among familiar individuals (z= 2,85; z= 2,97 and z= 2,08; p= 0.002, p= 0.0015 and p= 0.019, respectively, Jonckheere-Terpstra 1-tailed tests). Very significant differences confirmed these findings for the comparisons between the familiar (E) triads and the mixed (E+C) triads (U= 28, p<0.025; U= 24, p<0.01 and U= 33, p<0.05); for the comparisons between the mixed triads and the C triads of strangers (U= 23, p<0.01; U= 20, p= 0.005; U= 27, p<0.025); and, most significantly, for the comparisons between the familiar (E) triads and the C triads of strangers (U= 14, p<0.001; U= 12, p<0.001; U= 19, p<0.005).

From these experiments it can be concluded that forming groups according to the three conditions of social familiarity, of social familiarity together with social strangeness, and of social strangeness exclusively, results in physiological as well as in behavioural responses that together perfectly reflect these differences in degree of familiarity. These significant trends are found to parallel the three conditions of grouping: both plasma cortisol concentrations and reciprocal aggression are most elevated, moderately elevated, and least elevated in the conditions of total familiarity, intermediate familiarity, and total unfamiliarity, respectively. One would be inclined to relate these three concomitant factors to the possible perceptive processes that can in principle operate in the three conditions of grouping, i.e. respectively: detection of mutual strangeness among conspecifics; in the mixed triads, discrimination between a familiar and a strange conspecific for each one of the former littermates, plus the detection of two unfamiliar conspecifics two for the case of the stranger; recognition of mutual familiarity and of two conspecifics as particular individuals, identified as former distinct littermates. To the extent that it is correct, such interpretation would contribute to promote a cognitive approach to the problem of social stress. A similar approach has been proposed by Rushen (in press), when he concluded that assessment of fighting abilities as well as the psychological effect of immediate agonistic experiences of victory or defeat, are likely to explain why unfamiliar piglets of asymmetric body weight stop fighting after the 1st or the 2nd hour following their association as pair-members. In the present experiments, it is, rather, social or individual recognition that inhibit the initiation of fighting among conspecifics of symmetric body weights. It is, therefore, also very likely that the previous social experience of piglets as littermates determined how piglets assessed the fighting potential of a conspecific at the beginning of their encounter with familiar or strange group-members.

TABLE 7

Plasma cortisol concentrations (in ng/ml) of piglets tested in triads of strange individuals (C), or in mixed triads (E + C) of 2 familiar piglets ($e_1$, $e_2$) and 1 strange (c) individuals.

| Blood samples taken | E + C Triads N = 9 | | | C Triads N = 9 | | |
|---|---|---|---|---|---|---|
| | $e_1$, $e_2$ | c | Triad | $c_1$ | $c_2$ | $c_3$ |
| **Test - 24 hrs** | | | | | | |
| Medians | 32,5 | 33,9 | 32,8 | | 30,1 | |
| Means | 33,6 | 31,6 | 32,9 | | 31,6 | |
| **Test + 15-30 min** | | | | | | |
| Medians | 47,1 | 41,2 | 53,4 | | 51,0 | |
| Means | 50,7 | 42,8 | 48,1 | | 48,3 | |
| Comparisons | | | | | | |
| | | c | $p > 0.05$ | | C | |
| | | E + C | $p > 0.05$ | | C | |
| **Test + 2 hrs** | | | | | | |
| Medians | 26,2 | 33,6 | 29,7 | | 39,4 | |
| Means | 28,0 | 29,9 | 28,7 | | 40,1 | |
| Comparisons | | | | | | |
| | | c | $U = 14, p = 0.010$ | | C | |
| | | E + C | $U = 17, p = 0.025$ | | C | |

TABLE 8

Plasma cortisol concentrations (in ng/ml) of piglets tested in triads of familiar individuals (E), or of strange individuals (C), or in mixed triads (E + C) of 2 familiar ($e_1$, $e_2$) and 1 strange (c) individuals.

| Blood samples taken | E TRIADS<br>N = 20<br>$e_1$, $e_2$, $e_3$ | E + C TRIADS<br>N = 15<br>$e_1$, $e_2$ | <br><br>c | <br><br>Triad | C TRIADS<br>N = 12<br>$c_1$, $c_2$, $c_3$ |
|---|---|---|---|---|---|
| **Test - 24 hrs** | | | | | |
| Medians | 31,7 | 29,8 | 31,3 | 28,7 | 31,5 |
| Means | 34,2 | 31,7 | 30,4 | 31,3 | 33,2 |
| **Test + 15-30 min** | | | | | |
| Medians | 48,2 | 59,2 | 53,4 | 55,3 | 52,4 |
| Means | 47,6 | 56,9 | 52,6 | 55,5 | 55,0 |
| **Test + 2 hrs** | | | | | |
| Medians | 30,5 | 32,0 | 35,8 | 32,3 | 40,7 |
| Means | 29,8 | 31,3 | 32,5 | 31,7 | 41,9 |

TABLE 9

Statistical comparisons (U test) between the plasma cortisol concentrations recorded for triads of piglets grouped as familiar (E : $e_1$, $e_2$, $e_3$), as strange (C : $c_1$, $c_2$, $c_3$), or as 2 familiar ($e_1$, $e_2$) and 1 strange (c) individuals (E + C).

| Blood samples taken : | | 15-30 min after test | 2 hours after test |
|---|---|---|---|
| Comparisons | | | |
| E Triads | E + C Triads | | |
| n = 20 | n = 15 | | |
| $e_1$, $e_2$, $e_3$ | $e_1$, $e_2$ | p > 0.05 | p > 0.05 |
| $e_1$, $e_2$, $e_3$ | $e_1$, $e_2$, c | p > 0.05 | p > 0.05 |
| C Triads | E + C Triads | | |
| n = 12 | n = 15 | | |
| $c_1$, $c_2$, $c_3$ | c | p > 0.05 | U = 49, p = 0.025 |
| $c_1$, $c_2$, $c_3$ | $e_1$, $e_2$, c | p > 0.05 | U = 54, p $\leqslant$ 0.05 |
| E Triads | C Triads | | |
| n = 20 | n = 12 | | |
| $e_1$, $e_2$, $e_3$ | $c_1$, $c_2$, $c_3$ | p > 0.05 | U = 36, p < 0.001 |
| E + C Triads | | | |
| $e_1$, $e_2$    c | | | |
| n = 15    n = 15 | | p > 0.05 | p > 0.05 |

DISCUSSION

The extent to which the results summarized in this paper have decisively contributed to demonstrate specific effects of social stress must be discussed. Although the behaviours described can be ascribed to a variety of stressors acting in conjunction, the experimental paradigm presented here seems to have provided a clear-cut context for studying social stress. On the one hand, social stress was here assumed to be specifically induced by the properties of (a) conspecific(s) of a particular class, namely by strange individuals of same sex, and of very similar age, body weight and previous agonistic status. On the other hand, the behavioural changes that were assumed to specifically reflect stress, namely an increase of aggressive interactions, were related to hormonal measures traditionally considered to be relevant and reliable indicators of physiological stress, namely an increase in concentrations of plasma cortisol. And, as a general rule, it was indeed found that the levels of adrenocortical responses mirrored the behavioural changes, the two sets of measures being highest among strangers (C triads), of intermediate values among mixed groups of familiar and strange individuals (E+C triads), and lowest among familiar individuals (E triads). It could, therefore, be concluded that a significant increase in plasma cortisol concentrations indicated that more social stress was associated with a significant increase in reciprocal aggression, itself induced by social strangeness. But, because of the latter effect, it could not be asserted whether it was social strangeness or its correlate, increased aggression, that was the specific factor responsible for the elevation in the hormonal indices of stress. This point will be discussed first.

Social stress induced by the presence of strange conspecifics need not be always accompanied by aggressive behaviour following the encounters among strangers. There are many other possible behaviours by which strangers could express their psychological conflict and emotional disturbance. Further experiments should test if the presence of a stranger, e.g. only visually exposed, suffices to increase plasma cortisol concentrations in comparison to the visual exposure to familiar conspecifics of equivalent properties. The present experiments do not make it possible to know if stress was caused by the perception of social strangeness independently of the reciprocal aggression that was associated with the actual encounters between strangers. In the E triads, however, encounters were not followed by reciprocal aggression; even if the effect of behavioural contacts cannot be ruled out, since some unilateral agonistic interactions were observed, it is likely that the perception of familiar conspecifics reduced stress at the same time it inhibited aggressive responses. A similar conclusion cannot be drawn for the case of the mixed triads, because the perception of another familiar conspecific reduced aggressive interactions, but reciprocal aggression resulting from the encounters between the two familiar animals and the stranger eventually elevated the plasma cortisol concentrations of the former littermates. So, it is only among the members of the E triads that the presence of other familiar conspecifics might have specifically reduced social stress. Equivalently, individual recognition – and not just social discrimination between a familiar conspecific and a stranger – would be required to lower adrenocortical responses indicative of stress, whereas it also appears to inhibit the occurrence of aggression during encounters.

To conclude: in the present experiments, social stress could be considered to have been induced by the presence of strange and aggressive conspecifics encountered in an experimental situation susceptible of inducing environmental stress.

The second point to be emphasized is that aggressive interactions have been much more frequently recorded among strange conspecifics than among familiar ones. In principle, this result should not be surprising, especially in the case of the differences found between the triads formed exclusively from littermates (E triads) and those formed exclusively from members of different litters (C triads). The fact is, however, that in addition to the condition of grouping applied as experimental variable, all the animals could have manifested aggression or fear responses as a result of the overall stress caused by the test conditions. Generalized aggression could have been induced because animals of same sex and equilavent properties (age, body size and weight) were selected to form the three samples of triads. Besides, piglets of equivalent status in their respective hierarchies, excluding the animals of extreme dominant and subordinate ranks, were grouped ; such selection of animals with intermediate agonistic status very probably coincided with selecting animals of equivalent fighting tendency and ability. It is well known that such symmetries among potential opponents tend to induce reciprocal aggression. In contrast, animals whose biophysical properties and aggressive status strongly differ, very rarely fight and tend to readily establish dominance-submission relations on the basis of their detected asymmetries. As to generalized fear, it could have been induced in the present experiments by a variety of possible environmental stressors. Some of these correspond, for the piglets, to the following experiences.

Being taken out of their home pen, to which the members of a litter had become adapted after weaning.

Being separated from littermates, with whom they develop stable relationships and often establish personal bonds; agonistic interactions are rarely seen, whereas play, affiliative activities and synchronized behaviour become the general rule.

Being pushed, sometimes handled, to be forced to get out of their home pen and to be transferred into the experimental pen; sometimes, the piglets are disturbed by the intrusion of the experimenter into their pen and in all cases, the experimental transfers involve the sudden appearance of humans, often unfamiliar to the animals.

Being introduced into a new pen, perceived as unfamiliar. These possible stressors are even stronger in the industrial conditions of pig rearing, since littermates actually have to leave their native pens following weaning, are usually transferred into fattening pens located in different piggery houses, and often have to be transported into these totally unfamiliar environments, sometimes also very distant from their native piggery houses.

It is noteworthy that despite this overall environmental stress imposed in the present experiments, grouping the animals according to the 3 conditions selected for forming a triad exerted a very significant effect on both the levels of aggressive responses and those of plasma cortisol concentrations. In other words, the specific effect of social strangeness versus social familiarity was more important than the specific effect of being transferred into strange pens; equivalently, social stress was more consistent than environmental stress. This result is important insofar as adrenocortical response is also known to increase as a result of physical stress, such as handling and sudden changes in the normal environment. However, it must be added that social stress exerted robust effects only among the groups composed of strangers (C triads), and was consistently reduced only among the groups of familiar individuals, where individual recognition could operate (E triads). In the mixed triads, where just social recognition between a familiar and a strange conspecific could operate, the familiar animals showed agonistic as well as adrenocortical responses about as high as those recorded among their stranger opponents. This lack of significant differences could, as was mentioned earlier, be attributed to the fact that the presence and behaviour of the strange members of these triads induced aggression in the familiar animals, and vice-versa; but it could also be attributed to a more pronounced effect of overall environmental stress in these mixed triads. The same factor could account for the fact that in the mixed triads as well as in the C triads, formed with strangers, the specific effect of social stress on both aggression and cortisol concentrations declined after the 1st hour following the tests, to vanish after the 3rd or the 4th hour. Although it could be the case that social stress was maintained, and still more sustained among the strangers that formed these two samples of triads than among the familiar individuals of the E-triads, it may have become confused with the effects of overall environmental fear after these unacquainted animals started to react exclusively on the basis of their detected strangeness.

In the present experiments, a specific effect of social stress induced by association of strange piglets was probably facilitated by not using tranquillizers before the transfers (injections usually add to the overall physical stress mentioned above). Stress was also probably enhanced among strangers because as soon as animals perceive each other as unfamiliar, they start to manifest various fear responses (intense agitation and transpiration, accelerated respiration, defaecation, shrieks) which tend to be propagated to the other animals by contagion. These expressions of fear are sometimes still present when strangers initiate aggression, forcing the new partners either to engage in fighting or to respond by flights, in all cases by a dramatic increase in energy expenditure. Even when one opponent manages to readily dominate the other, the subordinate ceases to fight but has to resist severe aggression, and usually starts to show intense signs of fear.

To conclude: the present experiments have, fortunately, provided results that revealed a specific effect of stress induced by social strangeness, despite the general conditions of testing which inevitably involved many other possible causes of stress.

The last point to be discussed concerns the role of cognitive processes in the control of social stress.

There is no doubt, first, that aggressive responses are controlled by a perceptive process of social discrimination: detection of strange conspecifics induces or increases reciprocal aggression, and notably fights; in contrast, recognition of familiar conspecifics inhibits or decreases these aggressive interactions. Facilitation of aggression was found in the triads of strangers (C) as well as in the mixed triads, where the two familiar animals $e^1$ and $e^2$ were strangers for the animal c, and where the latter was a stranger for the former. Inhibition of aggression was found among the two familiar members of the mixed triads as well as among all members of the familiar E triads. As was previously discussed, individual recognition could only operate among the members of the E triads, where each animal probably discriminated between (i.e. identified) each of its group-member as a particular familiar conspecific. Simply social recognition could have operated in the mixed triads, where each familiar animal could discriminate between its familiar conspecific and the strange conspecific newly encountered. Since both the behavioural and the hormonal indicators of social stress were similarly increased by social strangeness, and decreased by social (or individual) recognition, it seems logical to conclude that social discrimination appeared to control social stress in the present experiments, enhancing it among strangers and alleviating it among former littermates. The question now raised is whether the strong differences recorded between plasma cortisol concentrations of pigs towards familiar and towards strange conspecifics may point to the existence of an adrenocortical correlate of social discrimination in agonistic contexts.

The results of the present experiments suggest that adrenocortical activity may be one of the neuroendocrine processes among the set of psychobiological mechanisms of social stress. Thus, adrenocortical activity could underlie the perceptive process that control the behavioural responses indicative of social stress, namely the detection of strange conspecifics soon followed by aggressive interactions and, conversely, the recognition of familiar conspecifics lowering or suppressing these interactions. Such hypothesis envisages that a certain neuroendocrine activity, typical of stress and of other emotional responses, may participate in the cognitive process that controls the nature, frequency and intensity of social behaviours.

So, in the present experiments, variations of plasma cortisol concentrations depending on whether group-members were familiar or strange, could be regarded as a physiological indicator of social discrimination, and not just as the hormonal measure according to which aggressive behaviour among strangers would reliably be considered as a relevant indicator of social stress. Changes in adrenocortical responses (e.g. plasma cortisol concentrations in pigs, or plasma corticosterone concentrations in domestic fowl) could be used in the future as a physiological measure that may strengthen the connection between emotion and social cognition in domestic animals. In this perspective, it would be informative to test the relation between adrenocortical responses and social recognition by recording behavioural patterns other than those observed in agonistic contexts.

REFERENCES

Arnone, M. and Dantzer, R. 1980. Does frustration induce aggression in pigs? Appl. Anim. Ethol. 6, 351-362.

Blecha, F., Pollman, D.S. and Nichols, D.A. 1985. Immunologic reactions of pigs regrouped at or near weaning. Am. J. Vet. Res. 46, 1934-1937.

Bryant, M.J. and Ewbank, R. 1972. Some effects of stocking rate and group size upon agonistic behaviour in groups of growing pigs. Br. Vet. J. 128, 64-70.

Craig, J.V., Biswas, D.K. and Guhl, A.M. 1969. Agonistic behaviour influenced by strangeness, crowding and heredity in female domestic fowl (Gallus gallus). Anim. Behav. 17, 498-506.

Ewbank, R. and Meese, G.B. 1971. Aggressive behaviour in groups of domesticated pigs on removal and return of individuals. Anim. Prod. 13, 685-693.

Ewbank, R., Meese, G.B. and Cox, J.E. 1974. Individual recognition and the dominance hierarchy in the domesticated pig. The role of sight. Anim. Behav. 22, 473-480.

Ewbank, R. and Bryant, M.J. 1972. Aggressive behaviour amongst groups of domesticated pigs kept at various stocking rates. Anim. Behav. 20, 21-28.

Fraser, D. 1974. The behaviour of growing pigs during experimental social encounters. J. Agric. Sci. Camb. 82, 147-163.

Fraser, D. and Rushen, J. 1987. Aggressive behaviour. In "Farm Animal Behaviour" (Ed. E.O.Price), Veterinary Clinics of North America. Vol.3, No 2, pp. 285-305.

Friend, T.H., Knabe, D.A. and Tanksley, T.D. 1983. Behaviour and performance of pigs grouped by three different methods at weaning. J. Anim. Sci. 57, 1406-1411.

Graves, H.B., Graves, K.L. and Sherritt, G.W. 1978. Social behaviour and growth of pigs following mixing during the growing-finishing period. Appl. Anim. Ethol. 4, 169-180.

Mc Bride, G., James, J.W. and Hodgens, N. 1964. Social behaviour of domestic animals. IV Growing pigs. Anim. Prod. 6, 129-139.

Mc Glone, J.J. 1985. A quantitative ethogram of aggressive and submissive behaviors in recently regrouped pigs. J. Anim. Sci. 61, 559-565.

Mc Glone, J.J. and Curtis, S.E. 1985. Behavior and performance of weaning pigs in pens equipped with hide areas. J. Anim. Sci. 60, 20-24.

Mc Glone, J.J. 1986. Influence of resources on pig aggression and dominance. Behav. Processes. 12, 135-144.

Mc Glone, J.J., Stansbury, W.F. and Tribble, L.F. 1986. Aerosolized 5x-androst-16-en-3-one reduced agonistic behaviour and temporarily improved performance of growing pigs. J. Anim. Sci. 63, 679-684.

Meese, G.B. and Ewbank, R. 1972. A note on instability of the dominance hierarchy and variations in levels of aggression within groups of fattening pigs. Anim. Prod. 14, 359-362.

Meese, G.B. and Ewbank, R. 1973. The establishment and nature of the dominance hierarchy in the domesticated pig. Anim. Behav. 21, 326-334.

Meese, G.B. and Baldwin, B.A. 1975. The effects of ablation of the olfactory bulbs on aggressive behaviour in pigs. Appl. Anim. Ethol. 1, 251-262.

Moss, B.W. 1978. Some observations on the activity and aggressive behaviour of pigs when penned prior to slaughter. Appl. Anim. Ethol. 4, 323-339.

Moss, B.W. 1980. The effects of mixing, transport and duration of lairage on carcass characteristics in commercial bacon weight pigs. J. Sci. Food. Agric. 31, 308-315.

Rushen, J. 1987. A difference in weight reduces fighting when unacquainted newly weaned pigs first meet. Can. J. Anim. Sci. 67, 951-960.

Rushen, J. in press. Assessment of fighting ability or simple habituation: what causes young pigs (Sus scrofa) to stop fighting? Aggressive Behav.

Rushen, J. and Pajor, E. 1987. Offence and defence in fights between young pigs (Sus scrofa). Aggressive Behav. 13, 329-346.

Warnier, A. and Zayan, R. (1985). Effects of confinement upon behavioural, hormonal responses and production indices in fattening pigs. In "Social Space for Domestic Animals" (Ed. R. Zayan), Martinus Nijhoff, Dordrecht, pp. 128-150.

Warriss, P.D. and Brown, S.N. 1985. The physiological responses to fighting in pigs and the consequences for meat quality. J. Sci. Food. Agric. 36, 87-92.

Wood-Gush, D.G.M. 1983. Elements of Ethology. Chapman and Hall, London.

Zayan, R. and Thinès, G. 1984. Individual recognition reducing social stress in piglets grouped for the start of the fattening period. In "Results of Pig Research" (Ed. IRSIA-IWONL), Brussels, pp. 169-180.

**SESSION IV : RESPONSE ASPECTS**

# NEUROENDOCRINE RESPONSES TO SOCIAL STRESS

Pierre Mormède

INRA-INSERM U259
Rue Camille Saint Saens
33077 Bordeaux Cedex, France

## ABSTRACT

Social factors can acutely trigger a "stress" response characterized by an increase of circulating corticosteroids and androgens in the male, and this response is modulated by behavioral characteristics of the situation such as the intensity of the interaction between animals and the outcome of the encounter (dominance vs. submission). However, this activation is frequently minimal or even absent, and in some conditions social factors can even protect the animals from otherwise stressful stimuli.

In normal stable conditions, the physiology of domestic animals does not seem to be influenced to a large extent by social factors, although experimental data are rather scarce. The role of social hierarchy can be demonstrated only when social strife is increased by crowding or by impairing the establishment of normal social bonds by rotating animals among different groups. These conditions lead to the emergence of endocrine changes and, in some cases, pathological consequences. These changes however are no longer non-specific but are quantitatively and qualitatively dependent upon many variables such as the genetic background, the structure of the group (mono- vs bi-sexual communities), the hierarchical position of the animal,... It is therefore misleading to speak of "social stress" as if it was a unitary phenomenon.

## NEUROENDOCRINE RESPONSES TO ENVIRONMENTAL FACTORS

When studying the neuroendocrine response to any kind of environmental factor, two aspects are important to consider: the influence of time and the behavioral action opportunities provided by the situation. Acute exposure of an animal to a so called "stressful" stimulus triggers a non-specific endocrine response, characterized by an activation of the adrenocortical axis, which can be demonstrated by an increase in circulating ACTH, ß-endorphin and corticosteroids, and of the sympathetic nervous system, with an increase in circulating catecholamines. This endocrine activation can be assessed by monitoring changes in blood hormone concentrations or responses of target organs (increase in blood pressure and heart rate, hyperglycemia, changes in white blood cell counts, ...). In the acute phase of the response, these changes are generally non specific since they result from an undifferentiated emotional arousal which initiates the alarm response (Mason, 1971). They can nevertheless be influenced by various parameters, the most important being related to the behavioral control opportunities allowed by the situation (Dantzer and Mormède, 1983).

Within a few hours, this acute response vanishes and the classical indexes of the stress response generally go back to basal levels or show little change compared to the usual variability of many of these parameters. It is therefore necessary to use different experimental approaches to demonstrate a long-term modification of the endocrine systems resulting from a persisting influence of the environmental factor under study. For the hypophyso-adrenocortical axis, dynamic tests of inhibition (by dexamethasone) and stimulation (by ACTH or acute stress) are best suited to study the functional state of the system (see for instance Mormède et al., 1984; Meunier-Salaun et al., 1987). Other functional indexes such as the existence of a circadian rhythm or circulating levels of corticosteroid binding globulin (negatively regulated by corticosteroids) are also very sensitive to environmental factors (Barnett et al., 1981). As far as the sympathetic nervous system is concerned, long-term stimulation has been shown in experimental animals to increase the activity of the enzymes involved in the metabolism of catecholamines (Axelrod et al., 1970). However, very few examples of this last type of approach are available in farm animals, except the pioneering studies of Stanton and Mueller (1976) on the effect of early weaning in pigs.

In chronic situations, the neuroendocrine pattern of response to environmental factors is no longer non specific but is dependent upon the physical and psychological characteristics of the situation and the outcome of behavioral attempts to gain control. This aspect is of the utmost importance in social studies, where the dominance/submission relationships determine the neuroendocrine response and therefore the possible pathological outcome of social strife (Henry and Stephens, 1977).

ACUTE ENDOCRINE RESPONSES TO SOCIAL STIMULATIONS

The most typical acute social stimulus is the mixing of animals from different social groups, as seen for instance when piglets are weaned, sorted by weight and mixed in groups with animals from different litters. Vigourous fighting follows during a few hours. The endocrine response to this situation has been studied in the laboratory by bringing together two unacquainted pigs (Arnone and Dantzer, 1980). It was shown that the encounter increases circulating corticosteroid levels but that the magnitude of the adrenocortical axis response is modulated by situational factors such as the intensity of the fight and the behavioral relationship between the animals, the increase of plasma cortisol being larger in the submissive animal compared to the dominant one. Social encounter also increases testosterone in the boar (Liptrap and Raeside, 1978). This has been best studied in the laboratory rat by Koolhaas *et al.* (1983), who also showed that the increase of circulating testosterone was larger in the dominant animal, and that the submissive rat displayed a long-lasting decrease of plasma testosterone levels after the social encounter. These changes may be important in modulating social behavior (Leshner, 1980; McGlone, 1984, 1985; McGlone *et al.*, 1987).

The release of corticosteroids in these social situations is nevertheless of limited magnitude, when compared to other situations such as the exposure to a novel environment (Dantzer and Mormède, 1981) or to an oestrus female (Liptrap and Raeside, 1978). In fact we were unable to demonstrate any change of plasma corticosteroid levels when calves from different social groups where mixed, although these animals showed the expected corticosteroid increase when introduced in a novel environment (Bouissou, Demurger and Mormède, unpublished results) Moreover, social factors such as the presence of another member of the social group, can reduce the neuroendocrine response to an otherwise stressful stimulus. For instance, frustration is a potent stimulus to activate the adrenocortical axis in pigs (Dantzer et al., 1980), but the activation in completely abolished when two acquainted pigs are submitted together to the experimental situation (Arnone and Dantzer, 1980). The protective effect of social bonds on the response to stressful stimuli has therefore to be considered.

Deprivation from social contact may also be considered as stressful. Total isolation has been shown to be a potent stimulus for cortisol release in sheep, although physical separation permitting limited social interactions had not such an effect (Parrot *et al.*, 1987). In pigs, subtle functional changes indicative of an increased activity of the adrenocortical axis (blunting of circadian rhythm of corticosteroids, decrease of plasma transcortin levels) have been described by Barnett *et al.* (1981) in pigs penned individuallly. Ratcliffe *et al.* (1969) have described pathological consequences of long-term isolation of young pigs, including behavioral withdrawal and an increased incidence of coronary arteriosclerosis. We have shown previously that individual housing of calves in wooden crates induced a long lasting stimulation of the adrenal cortex

(Mormède et al., 1983; Dantzer et al., 1983). Although this hypothesis has not been directly tested, it should be considered that social deprivation plays a major role in this effect. The same hypothesis has been put forward to explain the strong activational effect of the "novel environment test". However, it is frequently difficult to tell apart the influence of social isolation from other aspects of the situation, such as novelty which is by itself a very potent stimulus for behavioral activation and ACTH/corticosteroid secretion (Fraser, 1974; Dantzer, 1979).

## LONG-TERM SOCIAL STRESS - QUANTITATIVE ASPECTS

The interactions between animals observed during the early phase after grouping result in stable social relationships among members of the group and therefore, the response to acute social stress such as previously described is generally short-lived. Aggressive interactions last no more than a few hours (see for instance Meese and Ewbank, 1973; Friend et al., 1983, in pigs; Bouissou, 1974, in the bovine species). Three days after the grouping of young pigs we were unable to demonstrate any change in basal cortisol levels or in the response to a standardized stressor of transport stimulation, although social strife was increased by reducing the trough length (Dantzer and Mormède, 1981). In fact, it is quite difficult to induce long lasting social stress. Two situations have been used: crowding and rotating animals among groups, two situations where social strife is increased or where the establishment of normal social bonds is impaired.

Crowding is a complex notion integrating many different aspects of the competition between animals for environmental resources (Stokols, 1972; Siegel, 1976). It is not my purpose to consider each aspect separately (size of the group, population density, competition for food and shelter,...) since available endocrine data are rather limited and do not permit such an analysis. Although crowding was shown to increase the activity of the adrenal cortex in poultry, the magnitude of the effect is in fact rather limited (e.g. Siegel, 1960; Eskeland, 1978). In larger mammals, it is frequently necessary to use dynamic tests of adrenocortical function to demonstrate the existence of functional changes. In fattening pigs for instance, Meunier-Salaun et al. (1987) observed that a high stocking rate induced an escape of adrenocortical axis to dexamethasone blockade and an enhanced cortisol response to ACTH stimulation, two indexes characteristic of an overstimulated adrenocortical axis, although basal plasma levels of cortisol were unchanged. An increased cortisol response to ACTH stimulation was also observed by Friend *et al.* (1977, 1979) in dairy cows subjected to increased density and free stall competition.

Rotating the animals from one social group to the other impairs the establishment of stable relationships and maintain high levels of aggressive interactions among pen mates. This protocol has been commonly used to induce social strife in poultry (review in Siegel, 1976), quails (Edens, 1987) and laboratory rodents (Taylor *et al.*, 1987). Gross and Colmano (1971) selected chickens on the basis of their corticosterone response to this social challenge, showing that the intensity of the endocrine response was under genetic control. In an extensive series of studies, it was shown that both genetic factors and social environment influenced plasma corticosteroid levels and resistance to various pathogens. The sensitivity to parasites and to bacterial infections was reduced by high corticosterone levels, but it was the reverse for viral infections and tumors (Gross, 1976; Siegel, 1976). Increased social strife has been shown to be responsible for other pathological conditions such as high blood pressure in laboratory animals (Henry and Stephens, 1977).

## LONG-TERM SOCIAL STRESS - QUALITATIVE ASPECTS

The results of experiments in which social strife is increased by crowding or between-group rotation indicate that social pressure does not induce a non-specific "stress" response but that its neuroendocrine consequences are quantitatively but also qualitatively different according to many factors related to the situation and to the animal. Studies carried out in laboratory animals offer some perspectives on the nature of these factors.

One major environmental factor is the composition of the social group. Taylor *et al.* (1987) for instance demonstrated that rotating males among exclusively male groups was a potent activator of the adrenocortical axis function, as shown by heavier adrenals and higher plasma corticosteroid levels. On the other hand, the presence of females completely obscured the adrenocortical axis stimulation, in spite of a considerable increase in the level of aggressive behaviors, but conversely this was a potent stimulus for testosterone secretion.

The social status of an animal is a major determinant of its neuroendocrine response to social stress. With only a few exceptions, low social status (or submissive) males show an increased activity of the adrenocortical axis (as demonstrated by increased corticosteroid levels and enlarged adrenals), and an hypoactive hypophyso-gonadal axis (shown by reduced testosterone levels and accessory sex organ weights), whereas dominant males have an hyperactive sympathetic nervous system (increased activity of catecholamine synthesizing enzymes in adrenals and sympathetic ganglia) and an hyperactive hypophyso-gonadal axis. These differences may be spontaneous or induced by an acute stimulus (social encounter for instance).

These neuroendocrine characteristics of social ranking have been studied almost exclusively in male rodents and monkeys with a strong social order and/or in conditions of increased social strife (see for instance Brain, 1972; Henry and Stephens, 1977; Ely and Henry, 1978; Benton et al., 1978, in mice; Dijkstra et al., 1985, in rats; von Holst et al., 1983 in Tupaias; Eberhart et al., 1983 in talapoin monkeys; Sapolsky, 1982, 1986, in baboons). Much less data are available in females (Schuhr, 1987, in mice; Bowman et al., 1978, Batty et al., 1986 in talapoin monkeys). The few available data indicate that it is also true in farm animals (Eskeland, 1978, in hens; Farabollini, 1987, in rabbits), although negative results have also been published (Arave et al., 1977, in cows). More work is obviously necessary in this field.

CONCLUSION

The physiological consequences of social interactions between animals represent probably the best example to demonstrate the complex nature of neuroendocrine responses to environmental factors. The acute response is not an all or non phenomenon but is dependent on structural factors such as the genetic background and situational influences related to behavioral control of the situation. Long-term neuroendocrine consequences of social interactions are usually undetectable but can be seen when social strife is increased by crowding or rotation of the animals among different social groups. It is nevertheless frequently necessary to use dynamic testing to demonstrate the existence of these neuroendocrine changes. When present, these changes are profoundly influenced by many factors such as the genetic background, the structure of the group or the position of the animal in the social hierarchy. It is therefore misleading to speak of "social stress" as if it was a unitary phenomenon. Although acute social stimulation can induce a non-specific "stress" response, the global neuroendocrine response to social stimuli is by far more complex.

Many aspects of this response still need to be investigated, particularly in farm animals.

REFERENCES

Arave, C.W., Mickelsen, C.H., Lamb, R.C., Svejda, A.J. and Canfield, R.V. 1977. Effects of dominance rank changes, age, and body weight on plasma corticoids of mature dairy cattle. J. Anim. Sci., 60, 244-248.

Arnone, M. and Dantzer, R. 1980. Does frustration induce aggression in pigs? App. Anim. Ethol., 6, 351-362.

Axelrod, J., Mueller, R.A., Henry, J.P. and Stephens, P.M. 1970. Changes in enzymes involved in the biosynthesis and metabolism of noradrenaline and adrenaline after psychosocial stimulation. Nature, 225, 1059-60.

Barnett, J.L., Cronin, G.M. and Winfield, C.G. 1981. The effects of individual and group penning of pigs on total and free plasma corticosteroids and the maximum corticosteroid binding capacity. Gen. Comp. Endocr., 44, 219-225.

Batty, K.A., Herbert, J., Keverne, E.B. and Vellucci, S.V. 1986. Differences in blood levels of androgens in female talapoin monkeys related to their social status. Neuroendocrinology, 44, 347-354.

Benton, D., Goldsmith, J.F., Gamal-el-din, L., Brain, P.F. and Huckelbridge, F.H., 1978. Adrenal activity in isolated mice and mice of different social status. Physiol. Behav., 20, 459-464.

Bouissou, M.-F. 1974. Etablissement des relations de dominance-soumission chez les Bovins domestiques. II.- Rapidité et mode d'établissement. Ann. Biol. Anim. Bioch. Biophys., 14, 757-768.

Dowman, L.A., Dilley, S.R. and Keverne, E.B. 1978. Suppression of oestrogen-induced LH surges by social subordination in talapoin monkeys. Nature, 275, 56-58.

Brain, P.F. 1972. Endocrine and behavioral differences between dominant and subordinate male house mice housed in pairs. Psychon. Sci., 28, 260-262.

Dantzer, R. 1979. Intervention des endorphines dans le comportement émotionnel du porc. C.R. Acad. Sc. Paris, 289, 1299-1302.

Dantzer, R., Arnone, M. and Mormède, P. 1980. Effects of frustration on behavior and plasma corticosteroid levels in pigs. Physiol. Behav., 24, 1-4.

Dantzer, R. and Mormède, P. 1981. Can physiological criteria be used to assess welfare in pigs? In "The Welfare of Pigs" (Ed. W. Sybesma). Current Topics in Veterinary Medicine and Animal Science, vol. 11. (Martinus Nijhoff, The Hague). pp. 53-73.

Dantzer, R. and Mormède, P. 1983. Stress in farm animals: a need for reevaluation. J. Anim. Sci., 57, 6-18.

Dantzer, R., Mormède, P., Bluthé, R.-M. and Soissons, J. 1983. The effect of different housing conditions on behavioral and adrenocortical reactions in veal calves. Reprod. Nutr. Dévelop., 23, 501-508.

Dijkstra, H., Tilders, F.J.H. and Smelik, P.G. 1985. Hormonal aspects of chronic and acute social stress in hierarchical colonies. Vakblat Biologie, 65, 387-391.

Eberhart, J.A., Keverne, E.B. and Meller, R.E. 1983. Social influences on circulating levels of cortisol and prolactin in male talapoin monkeys. Physiol. Behav., 30, 361-369.

Edens, F.W. 1987. Manifestations of social stress in grouped japanese quail. Comp. Biochem. Physiol., 86A, 469-472.

Ely, D.L. and Henry, J.P. 1978. Neuroendocrine response patterns in dominant and subordinate mice. Horm. Behav., 10, 156-169.

Eskeland, B. 1978. Physiological criteria as indicator of welfare in hens under different systems of management, population density, social status and beak trimming. Scientific Reports of the Agricultural University of Norway, 57, 1-16.

Farabollini, F. 1987. Behavioral and endocrine aspects of dominance and submission in male rabbits. Aggressive Behavior, 13, 247-258.

Fraser, D. 1974. The vocalizations and other behaviour of growing pigs in an "open-field" test. App. Anim. Ethol., 1, 3-16.

Friend, T.H., Gwazdauskas, F.C. and Poland, C.E. 1979. Change in adrenal response from free stall competition. J. Dairy Sci., 62, 768-771.

Friend, T.H., Knabe, D.A. and Tanskley, T.D., Jr. 1983. Behavior and performance of pigs grouped by three different methods at weaning. J. Anim. Sci., 57, 1406-1411.

Friend, T.H., Polan, C.E., Gwazdauskas, F.C. and Heald, C.W. 1977. Adrenal glucocorticoid response to exogenous adrenocorticotropin mediated by density and social disruption in lactating cows. J. Dairy Sci., 60, 1958-63.

Gross, W.B. 1976. Plasma steroid tendency, social environment and Eimeria necatrix infection. Poultry Sci., 55, 1508-1512.

Gross, W.B. and Colmano, G. 1971. Effect of infectious agents on chickens selected for plasma corticosterone response to social stress. Poultry Sci., 50, 1213-1217.

Henry, J.P. and Stephens, P.M. 1977. "Stress, Health and the Social Environment. A Sociobiological Approach to Medicine". (Springer Verlag, New York).

Koolhaas, J.M., Schuurman, T. and Fokkema, D.S. 1983. Social behavior of rats as a model for the psychophysiology of hypertension. In "Biobehavioral Bases of Coronary Heart Disease" (Eds. T.M. Dembroski, T.H. Schmidt and G. Blümchen). (Karger, Basel). pp. 391-400.

Leshner, A.I. 1980. The interaction of experience and neuroendocrine factors in determining behavioral adaptations to aggression. In "Adaptative Capabilities of the Nervous System" (Eds. P.S. McConnell, G.J. Boer, H.J. Romijn, N.E. van de Poll and M.A. Corner). Progress in Brain Research, vol. 53. (Elsevier, Amsterdam). pp. 427-438.

Liptrap, R.M. and Raeside, J.I. 1978. A relationship between plasma concentrations of testosterone and corticosteroids during sexual and aggressive behaviour in the boar. J. Endocr., 76, 75-85.

Mason, J.W. 1971. A re-evaluation of the concept of "non-specificity" in stress theory. J. Psychiatr. Res., 8, 323-333.

McGlone, J.J. 1984. Aggressive and submissive behavior in young swine given exogenous ACTH. Dom. Anim. Endocr., 1, 319-321.

McGlone, J.J. 1985. Olfactory cues and pig agonistic behavior: evidence for a submissive pheromone. Physiol. Behav., 34, 195-198.

McGlone J.J., Curtis, S E and Banks, E.M. 1987. Evidence for aggression-modulating pheromones in prepuberal pigs. Behav. Neur. Biol., 47, 27-39.

Meese, G.B. and Ewbank, R. 1973. The establishment and nature of dominance hierarchy in the domesticated pig. Anim. Behav., 21, 326-334.

Meunier-Salaun, M.-C., Vantrimponte, M.N., Raab, A. and Dantzer R. 1987. Effect of floor area restriction upon performance, behavior and physiology of growing-finishing pigs. J. Anim. Sci., 64, 1371-1377.

Mormède, P., Bluthé, R.-M. and Dantzer, R. 1983. Neuroendocrine strategies for assessing welfare: application to calf management systems. In "Indicators Relevant to Farm Animal Welfare" (Ed. D. Smidt). (Martinus Nijhof, The Hague). pp. 39-46.

Mormède, P., Dantzer, R., Bluthé, R.-M. and Caritez, J.-C. 1984. Differences in adaptative abilities of three breeds of chinese pigs. Behavioral and neuroendocrine studies. Génét. Sélec. Evol., 16, 85-102.

Parrott, R.F., Thornton, S.N., Forsling, M.L. and Delaney, C.E. 1987. Endocrine and behavioural factors affecting water balance in sheep subjected to isolation stress. J. Endocr., 112, 305-310.

Ratcliffe, H.L., Luginbühl, H., Schnarr, W.R. and Chacko, K. 1969. Coronary arteriosclerosis in swine: evidence of a relation to behavior. J. Comp. Physiol. Psychol., 68, 385-392.

Sapolsky, R.M. 1982. The endocrine stress-response and social status in the wild baboon. Horm. Behav., 16, 279-292.

Sapolsky, R.M. 1986. Stress-induced elevation of testosterone concentrations in high ranking baboons: role of catecholamines. Endocrinology, 118, 1630-5.

Schuhr, B. 1987. Social structure and plasma corticosterone level in female albino mice. Physiol. Behav., 40, 689-693.

Siegel, H.S. 1960. Effect of population density on the pituitary-adrenal cortical axis of cockerels. Poultry Sci., 39, 500-510.

Siegel, P.B., 1976. Social behavior of the fowl. Poultry Sci., 55, 5-13.

Stanton, H.C. and Mueller, R.L. 1976. Sympathoadrenal neurochemistry and early weaning in swine. Amer. J. Vet. Res., 37, 779-783.

Stokols, D. 1972. On the distinction between density and crowding: some implications for future research. Psychol. Rev., 79, 275-277.

Taylor, G.T., Weiss, J. and Rupich, R. 1987. Male rat behavior, endocrinology and reproductive physiology in a mixed-sex, socially stressful colony. Physiol. Behav., 39, 429-433.

von Holst, D., Fuchs, E. and Stöhr, W. 1983. Physiological changes in male *Tupaia belangeri* under different types of social stress. In "Biobehavioral Bases of Coronary Heart Disease". (Eds. T.M. Dembroski, T.H. Schmidt and G. Blümchen). (Karger, Basel). pp. 382-390.

# PHYSIOLOGICAL RESPONSES TO ISOLATION IN SHEEP

R.F. Parrott

A.F.R.C. Institute of Animal Physiology and Genetics Research,
Cambridge Research Station, Babraham, Cambridge CB2 4AT, U.K.

ABSTRACT

Work is currently in progress to characterize the behavioural, endocrine, neuroendocrine and physiological mechanisms involved in the responses of sheep exposed to stress. Sheep are a highly social species and are particularly sensitive to the psychological stress induced by isolation. In this report, several experiments are described in which the endocrine and physiological effects of isolation stress have been examined. Isolation was found to have a greater stimulatory effect on cortisol release than handling or restraint, to elevate temporarily plasma noradrenaline concentrations, to have no effect on oxytocin release but to reduce transiently vasopressin secretion and to modify the release of prolactin. Isolation also reduced haematocrit and plasma osmolality, suggestive of an action producing plasma volume expansion. The response to isolation was partially reduced if the animals were provided with a mirror, indicating that the sight of other sheep may have stress-reducing properties. These findings indicate that the response of the sheep to acute stress is complex and that isolation provides a convenient means by which to study psychological stress in a farm animal species.

INTRODUCTION

Sheep are highly social animals and sensitive to changes in group structure. Separation from the flock is known to be particularly stressful (Kilgour & De Langen, 1970) and in a choice test it has been shown that sheep prefer human contact to restraint in the presence of other sheep and choose restraint in preference to isolation (Rushen, 1986). Observation of isolated sheep indicates that they find the experience aversive since they often make escape attempts and bleat repeatedly. Isolation stress, therefore, can be expected to have profound effects on the animal's physiology and, because no physical component is involved, this procedure provides an animal model of psychological stress in which a variety of endocrine and physiological responses can be conveniently measured. The sheep also is particularly suited for endocrine studies because blood can be humanely collected by jugular venepuncture, obviating the need for surgical catheterisation.

In the present report, recent work in which the endocrine and physiological responses of sheep to isolation stress have been investigated will be reviewed.

ISOLATION, VASOPRESSIN AND WATER BALANCE

Isolation (Kilgour & De Langen, 1970) and cool, humid conditions (Guerrini & Bertchinger, 1982) both provoke cortisol release in sheep. In the latter case, however, the increase in cortisol is coupled with decreases in water intake and urine production. This suggests that stress might have effects on water balance and vasopressin secretion in this species. However, although vasopressin has often been considered to be influenced by stress, the possibility that this may occur in the sheep has not been investigated. Accordingly, an experiment was designed to examine the effects of isolation stress on cortisol, vasopressin secretion and water balance in sheep (Parrott, Thornton, Forsling & Delaney, 1987).

Ten adult castrated rams were studied under two conditions, i.e., separation and isolation. Separation involved holding a sheep in a separate pen next to the communal enclosure housing its peers. Isolation involved transferring a sheep to a pen in a hut situated some distance from the sheep house. The experiment lasted 30h and, at various intervals during this time, blood samples (10ml) were collected by venepuncture and water intake was measured. The blood was centrifuged and the plasma stored at -20°C pending radioimmunoassay for cortisol and vasopressin and estimation of osmolality using an automatic micro-osmometer.

The endocrine responses of the sheep are shown in Table 1. Isolation produced significant increases in plasma cortisol, compared with separation, but no differences in vasopressin secretion were observed. However, there was an inverse correlation between cortisol and vasopressin that just failed to reach significance at the 5% level. These results, therefore, do not support the view that vasopressin is released during acute stress, although a different situation may occur in animals exposed to chronic stress.

The effects of isolation on water intake and plasma osmolality are indicated in Table 2. Isolation markedly inhibited drinking but did not

TABLE 1   Changes in cortisol and vasopressin during isolation

| | Experimental | Sampling time (h) | | | | | | | |
|---|---|---|---|---|---|---|---|---|---|
| | Condition | 0 | 2 | 4 | 6 | 24 | 26 | 28 | 30 |
| Cortisol nmol/l ($\bar{x}$±SEM) | Separation | 2.4 ±0.5 | 4.1 ±0.6 | 2.1 ±0.5 | 2.1 ±0.4 | 2.8 ±0.6 | 2.3 ±0.5 | 2.0 ±0.4 | 3.0 ±0.5 |
| | Isolation | 2.4 ±0.4 | 10.5 ±2.2 ** | 5.1 ±1.0 * | 3.3 ±1.1 | 5.4 ±0.9 ** | 6.9 ±1.8 * | 4.7 ±1.0 ** | 3.6 ±0.8 |
| Vasopressin pmol/l ($\bar{x}$±SEM) | Separation | 0.5 ±0.1 | 0.4 ±0.1 | 0.8 ±0.2 | 0.6 ±0.2 | 0.7 ±0.2 | 0.9 ±0.3 | 0.9 ±0.3 | 0.9 ±0.1 |
| | Isolation | 0.7 ±0.2 | 0.4 ±0.1 | 0.5 ±0.1 | 0.6 ±0.1 | 0.8 ±0.2 | 0.6 ±0.2 | 0.7 ±0.1 | 0.8 ±0.1 |

* $p < 0.05$, ** $p < 0.02, 0.01$ Separation v Isolation, two-tailed paired 't' test

result in any increase in plasma osmolality.  When the results were examined in greater detail, it was found that four sheep drank no water at all but still had normal plasma osmolalities at the end of the experiment.  This compares with an increase in plasma osmolality from 301.1±0.9 to 314.5±1.3 mosmol/kg ($\bar{x}$±SEM; $p < 0.001$) when the same sheep were deprived of water for 24h in a group.  Thus, these findings suggest that some form of plasma dilution occurs in sheep exposed to isolation stress.  However, when grouped sheep are deprived of both food and water for 24h, plasma osmolality also does not increase.  The conclusion from this would seem to be that grouped animals continue to feed during dehydration and, consequently, incur an osmotic penalty whereas isolated sheep presumably eat very little and their plasma osmolality does not

TABLE 2    Water intake and changes in osmolality during isolation

| | Experimental Condition | Sampling time (h) | | | | | | | |
|---|---|---|---|---|---|---|---|---|---|
| | | 0 | 2 | 4 | 6 | 24 | 26 | 28 | 30 |
| Cumulative Water Intake (ml) ($\bar{x}\pm$SEM) | Separation | - | 74 ±72 | 147 ±121 | 321 ±141 | 1900 ±327 | 2346 ±406 | 2699 ±491 | 3083 ±385 |
| | Isolation | - | 0 | 0 | 54 ±50 | 507 ±291 ** | 623 ±401 ** | 827 ±388 ** | 971 ±408 ** |
| Plasma osmolality Mosmol/kg ($\bar{x}\pm$SEM) | Separation | 304 ±1.5 | 307.2 ±1.4 | 304.5 ±1.3 | 303.9 ±1.4 | 306.3 ±1.4 | 306.0 ±1.6 | 304.6 ±1.6 | 303.9 ±1.7 |
| | Isolation | 305.3 ±1.7 | 304.0 ±1.6 | 302.6 ±1.4 | 304.0 ±1.1 | 304.4 ±1.5 | 304.3 ±1.2 | 303.6 ±1.3 | 303.6 ±1.2 |

** $p<0.01$ Separation v Isolation, two-tailed paired 't' test

change. However, although 24h water deprivation is not stressful in grouped sheep (Thornton, Parrott & Delaney, 1987), the effect of 24h food and water deprivation on plasma cortisol has not been measured. Thus, it seems that a possible effect of stress on water balance in sheep cannot, as yet, be excluded. There is evidence that gluco-corticoids produce plasma volume expansion in the rat (Moses, 1965), dog (Swingle, Da Vanzo, Glenister, Crossfield & Wagle, 1959) and man (Connell, Whitworth, Davies, Fraser, Kenyon, Richards & Lever, 1986) and cortisol has been found to facilitate transfer of water across the sheep placenta (Leake, Stegner, Palmer, Oakes & Fisher, 1984).

ISOLATION, RESTRAINT AND HANDLING

Although it would appear that vasopressin is not released during short-term isolation in sheep, the possibility that secretion might actually decrease when cortisol levels increase is of interest in view of the stimulatory action that vasopressin has on cortisol release (Antoni, 1986) and the evidence suggesting that glucocorticoids may inhibit vasopressin secretion (Raff, 1987). There is also a possibility that the other posterior pituitary hormone, oxytocin, may also be involved in the stress response of the sheep since a variety of stressors have been shown to induce oxytocin release in the rat (Gibbs, 1984,1986). Plasma concentrations of vasopressin and oxytocin were, therefore, determined in a further experiment in which sheep were subjected to 120 min. of isolation, restraint in a canvas sling, or handling (Parrott, Thornton & Robinson, 1988). Plasma levels of prolactin were also measured because there is evidence to suggest that this hormone is released by handling and restraint in sheep (Davis, 1972). In addition, estimations were made of haematocrit and osmolality to explore further the possibility that changes in fluid balance might occur during stress.

Eight adult castrated rams were subjected to, a control handling procedure when group housed, restraint in the presence of other sheep and, isolation, as previously described. Blood samples were collected by venepuncture during a 30 min. control period when the animals were in their group enclosure and at intervals during the 2h experimental period. Plasma concentrations of cortisol, prolactin, oxytocin and vasopressin were measured by radioimmunoassay, percentage packed cell volume of whole blood was estimated using an haematocrit reader and plasma osmolality was measured with a micro-osmometer.

The effects of the experimental procedures on plasma concentrations of cortisol and prolactin are indicated in Table 3. Handling produced a temporary increase in cortisol levels whereas the increase seen after restraint were more variable but persisted to the end of the experiment. The most dramatic and sustained increase in plasma cortisol was, however, produced by isolation. Prolactin concentrations declined during the period of handling and restraint, becoming significantly lower after 120 min., whereas there was no decrease observed during isolation. These results support previous behavioural observations on the aversive effects

TABLE 3   Changes in cortisol and prolactin during handling, restraint and isolation

| | Experimental Condition | Sampling time (min) | | | | | | |
| | | Pre-treatment | | Post-treatment | | | | |
| | | -60 | 0 | 5 | 15 | 30 | 60 | 120 |
|---|---|---|---|---|---|---|---|---|
| | Handling | 5.1 | 6.9 | 12.8 | 10.9 | 8.5 | 5.2 | 6.7 |
| | | ±0.5 | ±1.1 | ±1.3 | ±1.4 | ±1.0 | ±1.2 | ±1.2 |
| | | | | *** | ** | ** | | |
| Cortisol nmol/l ($\bar{x}\pm SEM$) | Restraint | 7.0 | 5.9 | 12.6 | 16.1 | 15.2 | 13.3 | 21.7 |
| | | ±1.3 | ±1.1 | ±3.4 | ±2.8 | ±3.5 | ±4.7 | ±4.4 |
| | | | | | ** | * | | ** |
| | Isolation | 5.3 | 7.5 | 12.7 | 22.7 | 25.0 | 12.9 | 23.4 |
| | | ±1.2 | ±1.2 | ±1.6 | ±3.7 | ±2.9 | ±0.8 | ±3.6 |
| | | | | ** | ** | *** | *** | ** |
| | Handling | 3.1 | 2.6 | 2.9 | 3.2 | 2.5 | 2.1 | 1.3 |
| | | ±0.8 | ±0.5 | ±0.6 | ±0.8 | ±0.4 | ±0.4 | ±0.2 |
| | | | | | | | | * |
| Prolactin nmol/l ($\bar{x}\pm SEM$) | Restraint | 2.4 | 3.1 | 3.7 | 2.7 | 2.6 | 1.8 | 1.1 |
| | | ±0.5 | ±0.6 | ±1.0 | ±0.6 | ±0.6 | ±0.4 | ±0.2 |
| | | | | | | | | ** |
| | Isolation | 1.7 | 2.5 | 2.5 | 2.3 | 2.2 | 2.4 | 2.4 |
| | | ±0.2 | ±0.6 | ±0.5 | ±0.5 | ±0.5 | ±0.5 | ±0.3 |

* $p < 0.05$, ** $p < 0.02$, 0.01, *** $p < 0.001$   Comparisons with pre-treatment mean, two-tailed paired 't' test

of isolation (Rushen, 1986) and indicate that isolation has a greater effect on cortisol release than restaint and that restaint has a larger effect than handling. The results also suggest that isolation stress may stimulate prolactin secretion in sheep.

TABLE 4    Changes in oxytocin and vasopressin during handling, restraint and isolation

| | Experi-mental Condition | Sampling time (min) | | | | | | |
| | | Pre-treatment | | Post-treatment | | | | |
| | | -60 | 0 | 5 | 15 | 30 | 60 | 120 |
|---|---|---|---|---|---|---|---|---|
| | Handling | 9.7 ±0.7 | 9.0 ±0.4 | 8.1 ±0.7 | 10.0 ±0.5 | 8.9 ±0.6 | 9.7 ±0.5 | 8.3 ±0.4 |
| Oxytocin pmol/l ($\bar{x}\pm$SEM) | Restraint | 10.9 ±0.6 | 9.2 ±0.9 | 8.4 ±0.7 * | 8.5 ±1.1 | 9.1 ±0.7 | 7.7 ±0.6 ** | 8.7 ±0.8 |
| | Isolation | 9.2 ±0.5 | 9.5 ±0.9 | 11.1 ±1.1 | 9.5 ±0.7 | 10.3 ±0.9 | 8.5 ±0.9 | 9.8 ±1.0 |
| | Handling | 2.3 ±0.6 | 1.9 ±0.3 | 1.7 ±0.2 | 1.6 ±0.2 | 1.5 ±0.2 | 1.8 ±0.5 | 1.3 ±0.2 |
| Vasopressin pmol/l ($\bar{x}\pm$SEM) | Restraint | 3.0 ±1.0 | 2.1 ±0.7 | 1.8 ±0.4 | 1.4 ±0.4 | 1.6 ±0.2 | 1.8 ±0.3 | 2.7 ±0.6 |
| | Isolation | 2.1 ±0.3 | 1.8 ±0.3 | 2.1 ±0.3 | 1.4 ±0.2 ** | 1.3 ±0.1 ** | 1.0 ±0.2 ** | 1.4 ±0.3 |

* $p<0.05$, ** $p<0.02$, 0.01 Comparisons with pre-treatment mean, two-tailed paired 't' test

Concentrations of posterior pituitary hormones during the experiment are given in Table 4. Oxytocin release was not elevated during any of the treatments but there were two occasions when levels were reduced during restraint. These results indicate that, in contrast to the rat (Gibbs, 1984, 1986), stress may not stimulate oxytocin release in sheep. Vasopressin secretion was also unaffected by handling and restraint, however a significant decrease that lasted for about 45 min was observed during isolation. Correlation analysis indicated that there was a significant ($p<0.01$) negative relationship between cortisol and vasopressin during isolation, confirming the trend found in the previous experiment. Since vasopressin synergises with corticotropin releasing hormone to stimulate the pituitary/adrenal axis in sheep (Redekopp, Livesey, Sadler & Donald, 1986), the present results may provide evidence for a complimentary negative feedback action of corticosteroids on vasopressin release.

The results relating to water balance are shown in Table 5. Under all experimental conditions, decreases in haematocrit and osmolality were observed. Note however, that the reductions were prolonged during restraint and isolation and that the main effects observed during handling coincided with the sampling times when plasma cortisol concentrations were significantly elevated (Table 3). This experiment was concerned with a shorter time period (2h) than the previous study (30h) and the results seem to indicate that there may be a temporary expansion of plasma volume in acutely stressed sheep that could be related in some way to enhanced cortisol secretion. This conclusion is supported by previous observations of decreases in haematocrit and electrolyte concentrations during handling in sheep (Fenwick & Green, 1986).

## MODIFICATION OF THE RESPONSE TO ISOLATION

The sense of vision is of particular importance to sheep (Hulet, Alexander & Hafez, 1975) and sheep respond to mirror images (Parrott, 1983) and photographs and films of other sheep (Franklin & Hutson, 1986). It was, therefore, considered that the lack of visual stimuli from conspecifies might be a factor involved in the stress response to isolation. Consequently, a study was carried out to investigate whether

TABLE 5   Changes in haematocrit and osmolality during handling, restraint and isolation

| | Experimental Condition | Pre-treatment | | Sampling time (min) Post-treatment | | | | |
|---|---|---|---|---|---|---|---|---|
| | | -60 | 0 | 5 | 15 | 30 | 60 | 120 |
| | Handling | 36.1 ±1.5 | 34.7 ±0.9 | 33.0 ±0.6 ** | 32.2 ±0.7 *** | 33.1 ±0.6 ** | 33.4 ±1.0 * | 33.8 ±0.7 * |
| Haematocrit %PCV ($\bar{x}\pm$SEM) | Restraint | 35.6 ±1.2 | 34.5 ±1.2 | 33.5 ±1.2 * | 31.9 ±0.8 ** | 31.8 ±1.0 ** | 30.5 ±0.7 *** | 31.5 ±0.8 *** |
| | Isolation | 34.7 ±0.9 | 33.3 ±0.9 | 35.0 ±1.4 | 32.6 ±0.9 * | 31.8 ±1.3 ** | 30.8 ±0.9 ** | 29.3 ±0.6 *** |
| | Handling | 301.6 ±1.9 | 299.5 ±1.5 | 298.1 ±1.5 ** | 296.8 ±1.7 ** | 297.5 ±1.3 ** | 298.2 ±1.7 | 299.0 ±1.4 |
| Plasma osmolality mosmol/kg ($\bar{x}\pm$SEM) | Restraint | 299.4 ±1.3 | 298.6 ±1.3 | 294.8 ±1.7 *** | 294.9 ±1.4 ** | 294.9 ±2.4 | 294.9 ±1.4 ** | 293.8 ±1.2 ** |
| | Isolation | 296.5 ±1.6 | 294.9 ±1.6 | 294.8 ±1.8 | 293.3 ±1.4 ** | 293.3 ±1.2 * | 291.5 ±1.8 ** | 293.1 ±1.7 ** |

* $p < 0.05$, ** $p < 0.02$, 0.01, *** $p < 0.001$ Comparisons with pre-treatment mean, two-tailed paired 't' test

providing isolated sheep with mirrors would reduce the magnitude of the resultant endocrine and physiological response (Parrott, Houpt & Misson, In Press).

Blood samples were taken by jugular venepuncture from 6 adult castrated rams before and during a 2h period of isolation. Two large reversible mirror panels were fixed in the isolation hut and each sheep

TABLE 6  Changes in costisol and prolactin during isolation with and without a mirror

| | Experimental Condition | Pre-treatment | | Sampling time (min) Post-treatment | | | | | |
|---|---|---|---|---|---|---|---|---|---|
| | | -15 | 0 | 15 | 30 | 45 | 60 | 75 | 90 | 105 |
| Cortisol nmol/l ($\bar{x}\pm$SEM) | No Mirror | 7.7 ±0.7 | 10.7 ±1.3 | 17.5 ±3.1 * | 16.6 ±3.9 | 13.5 ±1.3 ** | 12.9 ±0.9 ** | 13.5 ±1.8 | 15.3 ±1.5 ** | 15.5 ±2.0 * |
| | Mirror | 6.3 ±0.6 | 9.5 ±2.0 | 16.2 ±1.7 ** | 19.7 ±5.6 | 14.9 ±3.9 | 10.7 ±2.0 | 10.0 ±1.7 | 11.1 ±1.6 | 12.0 ±1.1 *** |
| Prolactin nmol/l ($\bar{x}\pm$SEM) | No Mirror | 0.15 ±0.08 | 0.48 ±0.20 | 0.40 ±0.13 | 0.80 ±0.40 | 0.73 ±0.48 | 0.60 ±0.33 | 1.07 ±0.60 | 1.64 ±1.07 | 1.28 ±0.44 |
| | Mirror | 0.19 ±0.09 | 0.30 ±0.06 | 0.28 ±0.13 | 0.33 ±0.12 | 0.32 ±0.15 | 0.48 ±0.15 | 0.36 ±0.20 | 0.51 ±0.29 | 0.56 ±0.34 |

* $p<0.05$, ** $p<02$, $0.01$, *** $p<0.001$ Comparisons with pre-treatment mean, two-tailed paired 't' test

was tested once under 'mirror' and 'no mirror' conditions. Testing was carried out in a counterbalanced order and behavioural observations were made of the sheep during isolation using a video-camera. Plasma obtained from the blood samples was analysed by radioimmunoassay for cortisol and prolactin and haematocrit and osmolality were estimated as previously described.

TABLE 7    Changes in hematocrit and osmolality during isolation with and without a mirror

| | Experi-mental Condition | Pre-treatment | | Sampling time (min) Post-treatment | | | | | | |
|---|---|---|---|---|---|---|---|---|---|---|
| | | -15 | 0 | 15 | 30 | 45 | 60 | 75 | 90 | 105 |
| Haem-atocrit % PCV ($\bar{x}$±SEM) | No Mirror | 37.1 ±0.9 | 37.5 ±1.6 | 37.6 ±1.5 | 37.0 ±2.4 | 34.3 ±1.8 ** | 33.2 ±1.8 ** | 32.7 ±1.6 *** | 32.7 ±2.1 ** | 33.6 ±2.0 * |
| | Mirror | 36.4 ±0.8 | 37.4 ±0.7 | 36.9 ±1.1 | 35.5 ±0.9 * | 33.8 ±1.4 | 33.5 ±1.2 ** | 33.2 ±1.4 * | 33.0 ±1.8 * | 32.9 ±1.1 ** |
| Plasma osmo-lality mosmol/kg ($\bar{x}$±SEM) | No Mirror | 304.1 ±1.3 | 301.4 ±0.7 | 301.4 ±1.2 | 300.5 ±1.1 * | 298.5 ±0.6 ** | 299.4 ±0.5 * | 298.9 ±0.5 ** | 300.2 ±0.9 | 300.2 ±0.6 |
| | Mirror | 301.5 ±2.9 | 304.9 ±3.3 | 300.2 ±1.8 | 301.4 ±2.9 ** | 298.3 ±2.0 * | 298.7 ±2.1 | 301.6 ±2.8 | 302.0 ±4.1 | 304.9 ±5.6 |

* p<0.05, ** p<0.02, 0.01, *** p<0.001 Comparisons with pre-treatment mean, two-tailed paired 't' test

The behavioural analysis indicated that the isolated sheep spent significantly (p<0.01) more time (75%) in the mirror quarter of the pen when the mirror was present and looked into the mirror for 50% of the time. Plasma cortisol concentrations were significantly elevated on more occasions in the 'no mirror' than the 'mirror' condition and differences between these two conditions were significant at the 75, 90 and 105 min sampling times (Table 6). Plasma prolactin levels were low because the experiment was carried out in the winter and no clear significant effects were found. However prolactin levels tended to increase with time and the final sample in the 'no mirror' condition was greater than the pre-treatment mean (p<0.05), but only at the one-tailed level.

The fluid balance results given in Table 7 show that decreases in haematocrit and osmolality occurred during isolation under both 'mirror' and 'no mirror' conditions. However the effects on osmolality, in particular, were more marked in the 'no mirror' condition. These findings again indicate an effect of acute stress on plasma volume and, taken together with the endocrine data presented above, suggest that the presence of a mirror during isolation did reduce the magnitude of the stress response. However, the effect was much less than had been anticipated, possibly because the mirror images were unfamiliar to the sheep.

## ISOLATION AND PLASMA CATECHOLAMINES

Little is known about the effects of stress on blood levels of catecholamines in ruminants. In the present study (Houpt, Kendrick, Parrott & De La Riva, 1988) blood was collected by jugular venepuncture from 6 castrated rams before and during isolation stress. After centrifugation, the plasma was stored at -30°C pending radioimmunoassay for cortisol and alumina extraction, followed by high performance liquid chromatography, to determine catecholamine content.

Plasma cortisol (nmol/l; $\bar{x}$=SEM) increased from 9.6±2.6 before isolation to 21.8±3.2, 16.5±2.8 and 18.9±2.6 at 10, 40 and 70 min after isolation, respectively (p<0.001, 0.05, 0.001; two-tailed paired 't' test). Plasma noradrenaline levels were increased 10 min after isolation (Table 8) but declined subsequently. There was no effect of isolation on adrenaline and dopamine levels.

TABLE 8    Changes in plasma catecholamines during isolation

| | Sampling time (min) | | | | |
| | Pre-treatment | | Post-treatment | | |
| | -30 | 0 | 10 | 40 | 70 |
|---|---|---|---|---|---|
| Noradrenaline | 111.2 | 200.2 | 429.5 | 285.3 | 103.8 |
| pg/ml ($\bar{x}\pm$SEM) | ±49.8 | ±103.8 | ±128.8 | ±78.0 | ±46.6 |
| | | | * | | |
| Adrenaline | 138.2 | 194.7 | 243.2 | 104.5 | 86.2 |
| pg/ml ($\bar{x}\pm$SEM) | ±18.4 | ±144.7 | ±67.9 | ±29.7 | ±26.3 |
| Dopamine | 61.5 | 44.7 | 78.3 | 43.0 | 32.5 |
| pg/ml ($\bar{x}\pm$SEM) | ±21.6 | ±14.0 | ±22.9 | ±15.9 | ±6.0 |

* $p < 0.05$ Comparison with pre-treatment mean, two-tailed paired 't' test

GENERAL DISCUSSION

A series of experiments have been described in which some of the
behavioural, endocrine and physiological responses of sheep to isolation
stress have been examined.  The results indicate that isolation is a very
effective psychological stress in this species and that the nature of the
responses produced are complex.

Sheep exposed to isolation stress showed reductions in water and
probably also food intake, although the latter was not directly measured.
Isolation produced a large and sustained increase in plasma cortisol
concentrations and, in agreement with previous behavioural findings
(Rushen, 1986), its effects were more severe than those of either
restraint or handling.  The increase in cortisol during isolation was
associated with a transient reduction in vasopressin secretion which may
represent a negative feedback effect at the level of the hypothalamus.
However, in contrast to the situation in rodents, none of the stressors
studied in these experiments stimulated the release of oxytocin.

Isolation also seemed to have a small effect on prolactin secretion but further studies are required to examine this in more detail. A temporary elevation of plasma noradrenaline concentration was also seen but there were no accompanying changes in adrenaline or dopamine. The decreases in haematocrit and osmolality that were observed during short term isolation suggest that there may be movement of water into the plasma during stress; this effect on plasma volume may be a response to unusually high circulating glucocorticoid levels. Finally, visual information in the form of reflected images modified the response to isolation stress, indicating that the sight of conspecifics may have stress-reducing properties in this highly social species.

In conclusion, because the social deprivation that isolation produces in the sheep is highly stressful, this procedure provides an ideal experimental model of psychological stress in a farm animal species.

REFERENCES


Antoni, F.A. 1986. Hypothalamic control of adrenocorticotropin secretion: advances since the discovery of 41-residue corticotropin- releasing factor. Endocr. Rev., 7, 351-378.
Connell, J.M.C., Whitworth, J.A., Davies, D.L., Fraser, R., Kenyon, C.J., Richards, A.M. and Lever, A.F. 1986. Changes in blood electrolytes, extracellular fluid volumes and atrial natriuretic peptide during development of ACTH and cortisol excess in man. J. Endocr., 108 (Suppl.), Abstract No. 154.
Davis, S.L. 1972. Plasma levels of prolactin, growth hormone and insulin in sheep following the infusion of arginine, leucine and phenylalanine. Endocrinol., 91, 549-555.
Fenwick, D.C. and Green, D.J. 1986. The effects of handling procedures, breed differences and treatment with lithium and dexamethasone on some blood parameters in sheep. Appl. Anim. Behav. Sci., 16, 39-47.
Franklin, J.R. and Hutson, G.D. 1982. Experiments on attracting sheep to move along a lane way. III Visual stimuli. Appl. Anim. Ethol., 8, 457-478.
Gibbs, D.M. 1984. Dissociation of oxytocin, vasopressin and corticotrophin secretion during different types of stress. Life Sci., 35, 487-491.
Gibbs, D.M. 1986. Stress-specific modulation of ACTH secretion of oxytocin. Neuroendocr. 42, 456-458.
Guerrini, V.H. and Bertchinger, H. 1982. Effect of ambient temperature and humidity on plasma cortisol in sheep. Brit. Vet. J. 138, 175-192.
Houpt, K.A., Kendrick, K.M., Parrott, R.F. and De La Riva, C.F. 1988. Catecholamine content of plasma and saliva in sheep exposed to psychological stress. Horm. Metab. Res., 20, 189-190.

Hulet, C.V., Alexander, G. and Hafez, E.S.E. 1975. The behaviour of sheep. In "The behaviour of domestic animals". (Ed. E.S.E. Hafez). (Baillere Tindall, London). pp246-294.

Kilgour, R. and de Langen, H. 1970. Stress in sheep resulting from management practices. Proc. New Zealand Soc. Anim. Prod., 30, 65-76.

Leake, R.D., Stegner, H., Palmer, S.N., Oakes, G.K. and Fisher, D.A. 1984. Cortisol facilitates ovine fetal/maternal water transfer. Pediat. Res., 18, 631-633.

Moses, A.M. 1965. Influence of the adrenal cortex on body water distribution in rats. Am. J. Physiol., 208, 662-665.

Parrott, R.F. 1983. A method for the quantification of butting activity in androgen-treated wethers. Appl. Anim. Ethol., 10, 319-324.

Parrott, R.F., Houpt, K.A. and Misson, B.H. Modification of the responses of sheep to isolation stress by the use of mirror panels. Appl. Anim. Behav. Sci. (In press).

Parrott, R.F., Thornton, S.N., Forsling, M.L. and Delaney, C.E. 1987. Endocrine and behavioural factors affecting water balance in sheep subjected to isolation stress. J. Endocr., 112, 305-310.

Parrott, R.F., Thornton, S.N. and Robinson, J.E. 1988. Endocrine responses to acute stress in castrated rams: no increase in oxytocin but evidence for an inverse relationship between cortisol and vasopressin. Acta Endocr., 117, 381-386.

Raff, H. 1987. Glucocorticoid inhibition of neurophypophysial vasopressin secretion. Am. J. Physiol., 252, R635-R644.

Redekopp, C., Livesey, J.H., Sadler, W. and Donald, R.A. 1986. The physiological significance of arginine vasopressin in potentiating the response to corticotrophin-releasing factor in sheep. J. Endocr., 108, 309-312.

Rushen, J. 1986. Aversion of sheep for handling treatments: paired choice studies. Appl. Anim. Behav. Sci., 16, 363-370.

Swingle, W.W., Da Vanzo, J.P., Glenister, D., Crossfield, H.C. and Wagle, C. 1959. Role of gluco- and mineralo-corticoids in salt and water metabolism of adrenalectomized dogs. Am. J. Physiol., 196, 283-293.

Thornton, S.N., Parrott, R.F. and Delaney, C.E. 1987. Differential responses of plasma oxytocin and vasopressin to dehydration in non-stressed sheep. Acta Endocr., 114, 519-523.

# EFFECTS OF BEAK-TRIMMING (AND CROWDING) UPON DEFEATHERING, ENERGETICS AND MORTALITY IN LAYING HENS

M. Herremans , R. Zayan[*], E. Decuypere

K.U.Leuven, Landbouwfaculteit, Labo Fysiologie der Huisdieren, Kardinaal
Mercierlaan 92,B-3030 Heverlee, Belgium
[*]Université de Louvain, Centre Albert Michotte, Biologie du Comportement,
1 Croix-du-Sud, B-1348 Louvain-La-Neuve, Belgium

ABSTRACT

Defeathering and mortality were studied in beak-trimmed and not beak-trimmed brown and white laying hens stocked at 3 or 4 per cage. Defeathering developed roughly exponentially in the course of the laying year. It was dramatically enhanced in not beak-trimmed hens and more severe in white than in brown hens. Density also greatly modified plumage condition, tetrads being clearly worse. In parallel to plumage condition there were influences on heat production, energetic efficiency and egg production. Defeathering resulted in an energetic stress such that especially the not beak-trimmed hens produced egg mass at the expense of body mass when kept at constant food intake. Energetics may govern the impact of social stress on production in laying hens, but it was apparent that primary effects of social stress were also present. The not beak-trimmed hens, and more so in tetrads, changed from their usual adaptive behaviour in such cage conditions to behaviour clearly detrimental to cage mates. Mortality rates followed plumage deterioration and might have reflected the ultimate consequence of behaviour interpreted to cause social stress.

INTRODUCTION

Beak-trimming is studied here as experimental variable because it is highly relevant to the problem of the welfare of laying hens. Great discussion exists as to whether beak-trimming should be practised to prevent cannibalism and social stress, or whether it should be forbidden for causing pain and physiological stress. Furthermore beak-trimming also affects defeathering caused by feather pecking; a reduction of defeathering following beak-trimming is reported by Hughes and Michie (1982).

Poor feathering increases heat production (Herreid and Kessel, 1967; Tullett et al., 1980; Lee et al., 1983; Herremans and Decuypere, 1986), shifts the thermoneutral zone to higher temperatures, and amplifies thermal responses at temperatures below this zone (Romijn, 1950; Richards, 1977; Nichelmann et al., 1978). As a consequence, maintenance requirements increase dramatically in poorly feathered hens, especially below 20°C (O'Neill and Jackson, 1974; Clark et al., 1975; Richards, 1977;

227

Johnson et al., 1978; Hill, 1980; Tauson and Svensson, 1980). Energy repartition, for a given energy intake, influences egg laying efficiency due to competition between components of the energy balance. Indeed, hens with lower heat production were found to produce more efficiently (Morrison and Leeson, 1978) and the more efficient hens in a flock had better plumage (Leeson and Morrison, 1978; Vanskike and Adams, 1983). Studies of energy balances showed the increases in energy loss caused by average defeathering under commercial battery cage conditions to be of economic importance (Herremans and Decuypere, 1988).

Defeathering has been ascribed to self-plucking (Hill, 1980; Hughes, 1980), to pecking between cage-mates (Hughes and Duncan, 1972; Hughes and Black, 1976; Preston, 1984) or between birds of adjacent cages (Hughes, 1978, 1980; Doyen and Zayan, 1984), and to wear caused by physical contact with cage walls and cage mates (Charles, 1976; Hughes, 1980, 1983, 1985).

Increased feather wear has repeatedly been reported when flock size and/or floor area per bird was increased (Kivimäe, 1976; Hughes and Duncan, 1972; Hughes and Black, 1974, 1976; Adams et al., 1978; Hill and Hunt, 1978; Tauson, 1980; Hughes, 1980; Ouart and Adams, 1982; Ramos et al., 1986; Koelkebeck et al., 1987).

All the above mentioned data point to an underlying relation between social stress and energetics. However, energetic consequences of chronic social stress in fowls hardly seem to have been comprehensively studied. Although this work presents a rather global account of some of the responses to social stress, the results reported allow to infer some physiological mechanisms by which chronic social stress can lead to loss of economic benefits.

## MATERIALS AND METHODS

Experiment 1 (Performed by M.H. and co-workers)

Warren SSL brown hybrid laying hens were housed 3 or 4 to each battery cage (with 600 $cm^2$/hen and 450 $cm^2$/hen respectively) under near commercial conditions. Half of the flock had been beak-trimmed during the first week of life (BT); the others had intact bills (NBT). From the start of egg laying onwards daily food intake was kept constant, initially to 120 g, but from week 9 on, to 130 g per hen day, which should be about ad lib for well feathered hens (Herremans et al., 1988). Houses were not heated to keep temperatures constant, but environmental temperature remained within 12-25°C range.

From cages in mirror symmetric position in the battery, 24 hens from each of the four conditions were used to study plumage deterioration after 9, 15, 26 and 33 weeks of laying. Hens had to be handled to obtain the index of body-plumage wear (IBPW), a criterion based on the estimation of the severity of the damage (how much of each feather is worn off, $w_i$) and the fraction of the area to which it occurred (how many of the feathers, $f_i$). Plumage deterioration ($FW_a$) was separately scored in six body-areas (pectoral, abdominal, femoral, dorsal, alar and capital, covering 75% of the total body-plumage weight) : $FW_a = \sum\limits_{i=1}^{n} f_i \times w_i$ . After correction for the mean body-plumage weight of the respective area in intact control hens ($G_a$), the estimation for the defeathering on the total body was calculated : $IBPW = \sum\limits_{a=1}^{6} G_a \times FW_a$ . Finally, IBPW was rescaled to range between 0-100, therefore to represent a %-estimate of defeathering (Herremans and Decuypere, 1987).

During the 7th month of laying, egg weight and rate of laying were followed in the whole flock (4x12 cages). Body weight was recorded individually after 7.5 months of laying. After 8 months of laying blood samples were quickly taken (within 45 secs) from the hens also studied for plumage condition (thus used to be handled), and corticosterone levels were determined by radioimmunoassay (commercial kits from Cambridge Medical Technology).

Samples of hens were removed (and not replaced) for metabolic trials in open circuit respiration chambers at environmental temperatures of 7°C (and also 14°C, 21°C and 28°C in some trials). Heat production was calculated from $O_2$ uptake and $CO_2$ production (Romijn and Lokhorst, 1961), which were measured by the diaferometer method, calibrated after Geers et al. (1978). After birds became used to the chambers during several days, energy balances were followed over a four day period with *ad libitum* access to food. Four cages were examined at the onset of the laying year. After 8 months of laying, 5 cages of beak-trimmed and 4 of not beak-trimmed triads, and 7 cages from the not beak-trimmed tetrads were removed for metabolic trials. The same cages from the last group were re-used after restoring a good plumage condition by artificial moulting. Afterwards, hens from two NBT tetrads were denuded by clipping off the feather cover, before they were resubmitted to metabolic trials.

Experiment 2 (performed by R.Z. and co-workers)

A second experiment concentrated in more detail on the effects of beak-trimming upon defeathering and mortality. Laying hens of two commercial strains (R = Rhode Island Red; W = White Leghorn) were subjected to 4 experimental treatments : some were precociously, and only once beak-trimmed at the age of 8 days (+-), according to the current practice in Belgian farms; some were again beak-trimmed at the age of 14 weeks (++); some were lately beak-trimmed for the first time at the age of 14 weeks (-+); some were never beak-trimmed (--).

All the birds were simultaneously and randomly housed in the same standard battery cages as in the first experiment (floor area = 1.800 cm$^2$), either in triads or in tetrads. In two consecutive series covering two years in total, 48 cages from each condition were studied for a period of 11 months. Because ethological causes of plumage deterioration had to be more clearly distinguished from the biophysical factors resulting in feather abrasion, a total number of 10 body areas was considered, instead of the 6 areas investigated in the first experiment. The following body areas were distinguished as a modification of the IBPW-method :

- The capital area was further differentiated in a) the capital tract and the upper part of the dorsal cervical tract, just below the comb (where subordinate hens are often pecked), and b) the lower dorsal cervical and ventral cervical tracts (the neck);
- The abdominal area was differentiated in a) the sternal tract (the belly), and b) the abdominal tract (the underbelly) together with the anal region (where birds may be severly pecked by pre-cannibalism);
- The dorsal area was differentiated in a) the interscapular tract or upper part of the back, and b) the lower part of the back (the rump) or dorsopelvic tract (which may be totally defeathered by pre-cannibalism);
- The tail-feathers or rectrices, (also typically pecked in case of cannibalism) were studied separately;
- The other areas (pectoral, alar, femoral) were the same as in the first experiment, except that the remiges were included in the alar area, and the crural tract in the femoral area.

The selected 10 body areas include about 95% of the total plumage of an intact hen.

For obvious ethical reasons, it was decided to stop observations on not beak-trimmed hens as soon as they were seen to become subjected to pre-cannibalism. It was, nevertheless, always checked that critical levels of defeathering in fact corresponded to observed intensive pecking, to consistent chasing behaviour or to preliminary bouts of killing behaviour in each cage where a bird was caught to be saved from death.

TABLE 1    Defeathering (in %) separately for each feather area studied, as related to age, beak-trimming and crowding in Warren hens kept in batteries (median of medians per cage; exp. 1).  One-tailed  Mann-Whitney-U  test  :    * P ≤ 0.05;    ** P ≤ 0.005; *** P ≤ 0.001.

Group-size n = 3 hens/cage,    floor area    600 cm$^2$/bird

| Nb weeks in cages | 9 | | 15 | | 26 | | 33 | |
|---|---|---|---|---|---|---|---|---|
| Beak-trimming : | + | - | + | - | + | - | + | - |
| **Body area** | | | | | | | | |
| Capital | 0 *** | 11 | 1 *** | 21 | 13 ** | 58 | 26 ** | 59 |
| Pectoral | 0 | 0 | 0 | 0 | 0 * | 2 | 0 * | 9 |
| Abdominal | 0 | 0 | 0 | 0 | 0 * | 3 | 0 * | 13 |
| Femoral | 0 | 0 | 0 | 0 | 0 | 0 | 0 | 5 |
| Dorsal | 0 | 0 | 0 | 0 | 0 | 0 | 6 | 19 |
| Alar | 0 | 0 | 0 * | 2 | 0 ** | 5 | 3 * | 16 |

Group-size n = 4 hens/cage,    floor area    450 cm$^2$/bird

| Nb weeks in cages | 9 | | 15 | | 26 | | 33 | |
|---|---|---|---|---|---|---|---|---|
| Beak-trimming : | + | - | + | - | + | - | + | - |
| **Body area** | | | | | | | | |
| Capital | 2 *** | 25 | 6 *** | 58 | 33 *** | 74 | 38 * | 71 |
| Pectoral | 0 | 0 | 0 * | 3 | 0 *** | 44 | 0 *** | 59 |
| Abdominal | 0 | 0 | 0 | 0 | 0 * | 13 | 0 ** | 14 |
| Femoral | 0 | 0 | 0 | 0 | 0 *** | 5 | 5 * | 19 |
| Dorsal | 0 | 0 | 0 * | 2 | 0 *** | 20 | 8 * | 25 |
| Alar | 0 | 0 | 0 * | 3 | 3 *** | 19 | 7 *** | 43 |

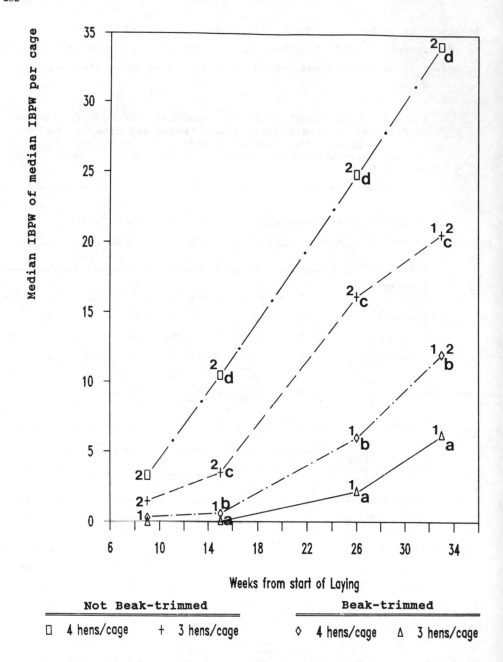

Fig. 1   Development of feather wear during the first year of laying in Warren hens kept in battery cages, as related to (precocious) beak-trimming and crowding (exp. 1) : 3 hens per cage (600 cm$^2$ /hen), 4 hens per cage (450 cm$^2$ /hen).   Statistics at the same age : different letter $P \leq 0.05$, different number $P \leq 0.0001$ (1-sided Mann-Whitney-U contrasts when Kruskal-Wallis ANOVA significant).

RESULTS

Experiment 1

Plumage deterioration developed roughly exponentially during the laying year, but the exact position of the curve was highly dependent on the management. Beak-trimming greatly reduced feather wear and the effect of beak-trimming was much more important than that of stocking rate (Fig. 1). Housing hens 3 to a cage resulted in significantly better plumage than housing 4 hens to a cage, but this is a mixed effect of the two density factors (group size and floor area per bird) that will not further be considered here. Feather wear did not develop simultaneously to the same extent in all body areas, but, although beak-trimming had great influence on the speed at which feather damage developed, the patterns of defeathering did not appear to differ much between beak-trimmed and not beak-trimmed hens (Table 1). The capital area was particularly vulnerable to defeathering, but especially in NBT hens (particularly in tetrads) the alar, dorsal and pectoral area also rapidly deteriorated.

After 8 months of laying, heat production was found increased in parallel to plumage deterioration, even at night when interaction from activity is absent (Fig.2). In these new conditions in the respiration chambers social interaction was not the most important factor to influence heat production. This can be judged from the parallel increase in heat production during the light and dark periods : increases in heat production seem to represent mainly thermoregulatory responses (Fig. 2; Table 2A). When compared to controls, plumage deterioration up to about 15-20% seems not to have had dramatic energetic impact under ad lib feeding conditions, even at 7°C (Table 2A, Figs. 2 and 3; compare also to Tullett et al, 1980). Restoring plumage condition by artificial moulting restored heat production almost to control values, but artificial denudation had dramatic impact, especially at lower temperature (Fig. 2). However, these metabolic experiments were performed in ad lib feeding conditions; thus, levels of heat production could have been influenced by different levels of energy intake. Energy intake, in turn, could have influenced egg production, thus also heat production.

A more complete picture of energy efficiency is found in the XY-plot of energy retention (eggs or body-weight gain) against metabolizable energy intake (Fig. 3). Although data are limited and scattered, it is clear that in general, the better the plumage, the more efficient the birds were (the more to the upper and left side of the figure), independently of the level of food intake.

234

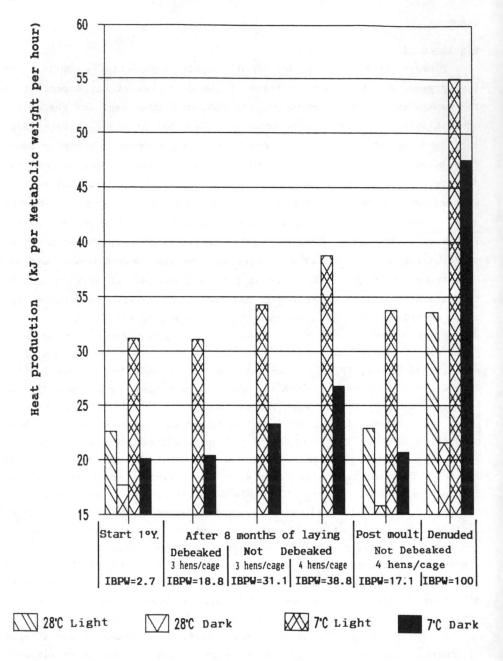

Fig. 2 Heat production in the light and dark at 7°C (and 28°C) in Warren hens as a function of %-plumage degradation (IBPW) related to (precocious) beak-trimming and crowding, or following artificial manipulation (exp. 1).

TABLE 2A    Effects of beak-trimming (1st week of life) and plumage deterioration on production criteria and heat production in Warren SSL hens transferred to respiration chambers (exp. 1).    (Controls were removed from the batteries at the onset of the experiment, kept individually and submitted to metabolic trials during weeks 12-16). Variables underlined are represented by medians, otherwise means presented.    "Weeks" refer to the time already spent in batteries.

Controls (N=6 hens; Median IBPW = 2.7)

| Environmental temperature | 7°C | 14°C | 21°C | 28°C |
|---|---|---|---|---|
| Food Intake (g) | 141 | 136 | 138 | 111 |
| Eggmass (g) | 62.4 | 65.8 | 62.0 | 62.5 |
| Heat Production (kJ per kg$^{3/4}$) | | | | |
|     Light (16 h) | 31.6 | 29.0 | 26.7 | 23.4 |
|     Dark (8 h) | 20.4 | 20.2 | 19.8 | 18.6 |

Week 42-52 : (7°C)

| Density | 3 hens per cage 600 cm$^2$ per hen | | 4 hens per cage 450 cm$^2$ per hen | |
|---|---|---|---|---|
| Beak-trimming : | + | - | + | - |
| Sample size | 5 cages | 5 cages | - | 7 cages |
| IBPW (%) | 18.8 | 31.1 | | 38.8 |
| Food Intake (g) | 126 | 133 | | 146 |
| Eggmass (g/hd) | 60.4 | 55.1 | | 60.1 |
| Heat production | | | | |
|     Light (16 h) | 31.1 | 34.3 | | 38.8 |
|     Dark (8 h) | 20.4 | 23.3 | | 26.8 |

Energetic effects found in respiration chambers were also reflected in the production criteria of hens kept under commercial conditions. Beak-trimmed hens remained all in rather good plumage condition and they produced at high rate, independent of crowding (89.2% and 90.5%), resulting in similarly good egg-mass (58.5 g/hd) and food conversion (2.22; Table 2B).    Not beak-trimmed triads showed slightly affected production (84.5%, 55.0 g/hd and FC of 2.36), in accordance to energetic results (Figs. 2 and 3).    As could be expected from Figs. 2 and 3, the group of not beak-trimmed tetrads had dramatically reduced egg production (53.8%, 34.6 g/hd) and, from the economic point of view detrimental food conversion (3.76).

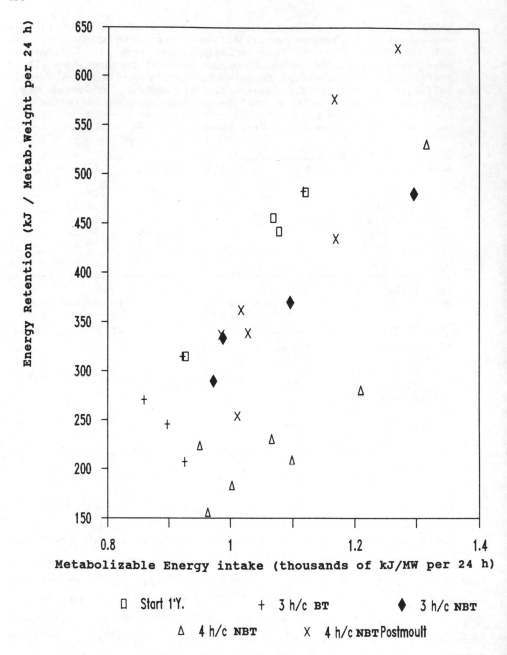

Fig. 3   Net-energy retention in relation to (apparent) metabolizable energy intake as a function of plumage condition in Warren hens at 7°C (exp. 1) : start 1° year IBPW = 2.7; after 8 months, BT triads IBPW = 18.8; NBT triads IBPW = 31.1; NBT tetrads IBPW = 38.8; post moult, NBT tetrads IBPW = 17.1.

TABLE 2B    Effects of beak-trimming (1st week of life) on plumage deterioration and production criteria in Warren SSL hens kept in batteries; food intake limited at 130 g/henday (exp. 1).  N = 8 cages per group, except for week 29-32 in not beak-trimmed hens (N=12 cages).   One-sided Mann-Whitney-U contrasts when Kruskal-Wallis 1-factor ANOVA significant : * P ≤ 0.05,   ** P ≤ 0.01,   *** P ≤ 0.001.

| Density | 3 hens per cage 600 cm$^2$ per hen | | | 4 hens per cage 450 cm$^2$ per hen | | |
|---|---|---|---|---|---|---|
| Beak trimming : | + | | - | + | | - |
| **Week 26 :** | | | | | | |
| IBPW (%) | 2.2 | *** | 16.2 | * 6.0 | *** | 24.9 |
| **Week 29-32 :** | | | | | | |
| Rate of Laying (%) *(1)* | 89.2 | NS | 84.5 | 90.5 | *** | 53.8 |
| Eggweight (g) *(2)* | 65.6 | NS | 65.1 | ** 64.7 | NS | 64.3 |
| Eggmass (g/hd) *(3)* | 58.5 | > | 55.0 | 58.5 | >> | 34.6 |
| FC *(3)* | 2.22 | < | 2.36 | 2.22 | << | 3.76 |
| **Week 33 :** | | | | | | |
| Body Weight (kg) | 2.16 | ** | 1.93 | * 2.03 | ** | 1.84 |
| IBPW (%) | 6.3 | ** | 20.6 | * 12.0 | ** | 34.2 |

*(1)*  statistically tested on the total number of eggs per cage during 4 weeks (sample size = number of cages);
*(2)*  statistically tested on the total weight per sample of 30 eggs (sample sizes = 13, 25, 21, 21 respectively);
*(3)*  4 week period considered *in toto* ; no statistics possible, but > < indicate differences considered of economical importance.

However, despite the lower egg output in NBT tetrads, there was not a compensatory body-weight gain either : in fact, the reduced efficiency affected both egg mass produced and body condition (Fig. 4; Table 2B). The NBT tetrads needed so much energy to compensate the losses due to reduced insulation, that they could not maintain high laying rates, but also depleted body-conditions to remain in energetic equilibrium at constant energy uptake.   Although some of the other groups had egg productions rather similar to the beak-trimmed triads, they did so at the expense of body condition (Fig. 4).   Reduction of organs when egg-laying ceases (the liver and the reproductive tract in particular) may have interfered to a very limited extent in body-weight losses, as presented in Fig. 4.   Especially in the NBT tetrads, which had the lowest egg production, a number of hens probably simply stopped laying.

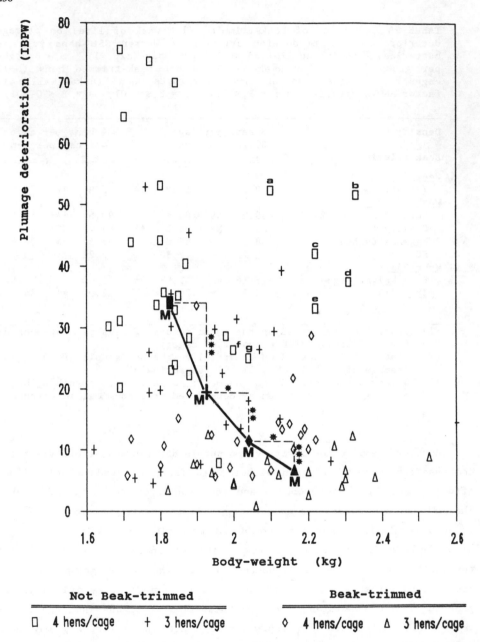

Fig. 4   Relation between plumage degradation and body-weight in Warren hens, after 7.5 months of laying at constant food intake.   Differences in feathering caused by interactions of (precocious) beak-trimming and crowding (exp. 1).   M = median for X and Y ; Total Spearman rankcorrelation $r_s$ = -0.27,   P < 0.005.   Contrasts between groups : 2-sided Mann-Whitney-U when Kruskal-Wallis significant : * P ≤ 0.05, ** P ≤ 0.01, *** P ≤ 0.001.   a,b,c,d,e,f,g indicate the heaviest hen in each cage of the NBT tetrads.

Experiment 2

In the cages with 3 hens of the R strain, both mortality and defeathering were reduced when hens had been precociously beak-trimmed; they critically increased when hens had not been initially beak-trimmed, to reach a dramatic rate when hens had not been beak-trimmed at all (Table 3). A similar trend was found in the same R hens when housed 4 birds to a cage, but mortality and defeathering were more pronounced at this higher

TABLE 3    Mortality (%) and mean defeathering scores after 11 months in battery cages. Hens beak-trimmed (+) or not (-) during the 1st week of life, and/or subsequently at the age of 14 weeks (exp. 2).

**R (Rhode Island Red) hens**

| n = 3 birds per cage | Floor area : 600 cm$^2$/bird | | | |
|---|---|---|---|---|
| Beak-trimming : | + − | + + | − + | − − |
| Mortality : | 3,4 | 2,8 | 4,8 | 8,3 |
| Defeathering : | | | | |
| — total body | 13,3 | 14,7 | 21,3 | 33,7 |
| — A + C + D areas | 15,1 | 16,8 | 29,8 | 59,4 |

| n = 4 birds per cage | Floor area : 450 cm$^2$/bird | | | |
|---|---|---|---|---|
| Beak-trimming : | + − | + + | − + | − − |
| Mortality : | 3,6 | 6,3 | 9,4 | 13,5 |
| Defeathering : | | | | |
| — total body | 21,2 | 22,8 | 38,6 | 48,2 |
| — A + C + D areas | 22,5 | 23,4 | 53,5 | 73,8 |

| n = 3 ≠ n = 4 comparisons | | | | |
|---|---|---|---|---|
| Mortality : | — | * | * * | * * |
| Defeathering : | * * | * * | * * * | * * * |

A + C + D areas : Abdominal-anal, Caudal, Dorsopelvic tracts
*,   **,   ***   :    p ⩽ 0.05, p ⩽ 0.01, p ⩽ 0.005

density. The difference between the two density conditions is very significant only when hens were not initially beak-trimmed, a result that cannot equivocally be attributed to group-size, since floor area per bird was also reduced in tetrads (450 $cm^2$ instead of 600 $cm^2$).

As can be seen from Table 4, the results found with the lighter strain W permit to draw similar conclusions. As a general rule, mortality and state of defeathering were clearly (and very significantly, $P<0.005$)

TABLE 4   Mortality (%) and mean defeathering scores after 11 months in battery cages.  Hens beak-trimmed (+) or not (-) during the 1st week of life, and/or subsequently at the age of 14 weeks (exp. 2).

**W (White Leghorn) hens**

| n = 3 birds per cage | Floor area : 600 cm²/bird | | | |
|---|---|---|---|---|
| Beak-trimming : | + − | + + | − + | − − |
| Mortality : | 4,2 | 6,2 | 9,6 | 17,3 |
| Defeathering : | | | | |
| — total body | 11,4 | 20,7 | 31,6 | 55,3 |
| — A + C + D areas | 12,7 | 19,3 | 48,3 | 68,6 |

| n = 4 birds per cage | Floor area : 450 cm²/bird | | | |
|---|---|---|---|---|
| Beak-trimming : | + − | + + | − + | − − |
| Mortality : | 5,5 | 9,9 | 14,6 | 28,6 |
| Defeathering : | | | | |
| — total body | 17,8 | 32,4 | 48,7 | 61,4 |
| — A + C + D areas | 20,2 | 34,3 | 62,5 | 79,7 |

| n = 3 ≠ n = 4 comparisons | | | | |
|---|---|---|---|---|
| Mortality : | — | * | * * | * * |
| Defeathering : | * * | * * | * * * | * * |

A + C + D areas : Abdominal-anal, Caudal, Dorsopelvic tracts
*,   * *,   * * *   :   $p \leqslant 0.05$, $p \leqslant 0.01$, $p \leqslant 0.005$

higher in the W hens, the only exception being found in the birds which had only been subjected to early beak-trimming.

A rough estimation of the significant differences between the four independent samples (of 48 cages of each strain in each cage density) can be provided by a Kruskal-Wallis 1-way test (KW-values for dF=3). However, a Jonckheere-Terpstra test for ordered alternatives will more specifically reveal the direction of such differences, namely by testing the significance level of a transitive trend among the samples (z-values for k=4). Such transitivity is actually represented by mortality and defeathering, being : least in the (+-) condition (hens only precociously beak-trimmed); slightly higher in the (++) condition; more pronounced in the hens only lately beak-trimmed (-+); most pronounced in the never beak-trimmed hens (--). Under such basis, the two extreme conditions (+-) and (--) could be expected to differ very significantly (Mann-Whitney U test). The result can be summarized as follows :

- The hypothesis of overall significant differences between the 4 samples was very strongly confirmed. The following results were found for mortality and defeathering, respectively : in the R triads, $P<0.01$ and $P<0.005$; in the R tetrads, $P<0.001$ and $P<0.01$; in the W triads and tetrads, $P<0.001$ for both variables in each condition.
- The hypothesis of a significantly increasing trend was confirmed in all cases : in the R triads (mortality $P<0.05$, defeathering $P<0.001$); in the R tetrads (mortality $P<0.001$, defeathering $P<0.01$); in the W triads and tetrads ($P<0.001$ for both variables in each condition).
- As could be predicted, mortality and defeathering showed the most spec-tacular significant differences between the (+-) and the (--) samples (all z-values at $P<0.0001$ level in U comparisons), correspon-ding in the former to the most favourable condition for the hens and, in the latter, to such unfavourable conditions that should better be avoided.

The behavioural interpretation of the results requires to distinguish initially beak-trimmed birds from not initially beak-trimmed hens. Only among the latter an extremely aggressive behaviour was observed, usually after 5 months in the battery cages. This chasing behaviour consisted of continuous pecking, often preceded by jumps, addressed to repeatedly fleeing and screeming cagemate(s); this behaviour caused severe defeathering and eventually degenerated into killing behaviour and proper cannibalism. Although such pre-cannibalistic behaviour was occasionnally observed in initially beak-trimmed hens kept in tetrads, it was systematically observed, and was significantly more frequent among the members of tetrads not initially beak-trimmed, particularly in the hens of the W strain. In triads, mortality was never caused by killing behaviour in the initially beak-trimmed birds, whereas a great majority of the initially not beak-trimmed birds which had reached a state of strong defeathering would have been killed if they had not been taken out of their cage (they were observed to be strongly chased by at least one cagemate, and sometimes started to present injuries unnoticed to the experimenter). The defeathering scores recorded for the abdominal-anal, caudal, and dorsopelvic tracts, confirm that the absence of initial beak-trimming leads to feather losses caused by feather pecking and pre-cannibalistic behaviour.

DISCUSSION

The feather deterioration reported here did not discern between abrasive wear and feathers pecked out, but only gives an overall estimate. Part of it seems caused by pecking (especially on the nape, back, anal and caudal region), and part of it seems due to abrasive wear (lower neck, breast, belly, wings, thigh; Table 5). Wear itself may be the direct or indirect result of increased social tension : reduced physical space simply increases the chances of wear, but more frequent and more severe social interactions also affect the frequency and intensity of wear (e.g. by increased activity). Furthermore, reduced space and/or increased social tension may indirectly affect the disposition to feather wear by behavioural changes : reduced physical space and increased social stress can reduce the time and quality of the preening behaviour, which, becoming insufficient, makes the feathers more susceptible to wear (Lucas and Stettenheim, 1972).

The energetic implications seem so important that they can be seen as a governing system : elevated social stress leads to changes which affect plumage condition, which, in turn, influences energy loss and repartition between components of the energy balance. Too severe energy loss can cause body-weight loss, so much that egg-laying stops and therefore chronic "spontaneous" moulting occurs in at least part of the flock. This obviously results in dramatically reduced economic benefits. Because in such a process several animals change from a reproductive to a survival state, dramatic endocrinological and concomitant behavioural changes can also be expected.

TABLE 5    Hypothetic main causes of feather degradation in several body areas of hens caged in batteries.

|  |  | Major causes of defeathering | |
| --- | --- | :---: | :---: |
| Body Area / | Tracts | wear | pecks |
| Head | capital<br>upper dorsal cervical |  | * |
| Neck | lower dorsal cervical<br>ventral cervical | * |  |
| Breast | pectoral | * |  |
| Belly | sternal | * |  |
| Abdomen | Abdominal | * | * |
| Cloaca | cloacal circlet |  | * |
| Wing | humeral, posthumeral,<br>coverts, remiges | * |  |
| Thigh | femoral, crural | * | * |
| Back | interscapular |  | * |
| Rump | dorsopelvic |  | * |
| Tail | caudal |  | * |

It can, however, be argued that it goes right the other way around · social stress might directly cause hormonal changes (elevated corticosterone, catecholamines) resulting in enhanced metabolism, which lead to increased heat loss, merely facilitated by the parallel feather deterioration.    Chronic hormonal changes associated with stress might break themselves directly through the pituitary-ovarian hormonal interaction related to egg-laying state.    It has been shown in mammals that a hyperadrenal state depresses ovarian function possibly by a direct antagonism with LH release (Li and Wagner, 1983a,b).    However, corticosterone levels (as they were here determined) did not differ according to conditions, neither were they individually related to plumage condition.    So, if this last hypothesis is the better one, then at least it could be concluded that corticosterone (in the present experiment) was not a good parameter to assay long term chronic social stress.    A similar conclusion follows from the report of Cunningham et al. (1988).

However, in contrast to the short term results from the respiration chambers, in battery conditions with limited food intake, long term changes in production were already clear at a state of defeathering of ca.

16% (Table 2B), and they became already dramatical at an IBPW of 30%. At week 22-23, thus before the main increase in plumage deterioration, a preliminary sample of production criteria recorded during 11 days did not reveal such dramatically low laying performances in the not beak-trimmed tetrads (79.4% laying, 51.6 g/hd aggmass, 2.52 food conversion).

That a more ethological process was also involved can be asserted because increased defeathering could be unequivocally interpreted as an effect of not beak-trimming the hens at an early age. In addition, the experimental variable was found to simultaneously correspond to the development of behaviour detrimental to cagemates : first, feather-pecking, in conjunction with direct agonistic interactions (pecks causing avoidances); subsequently, pre-cannibalistic behaviour (chasing, by means of pecks and jumps causing flights and shrieks) which, if not interrupted by the experimenter, would cause wounds, induce killing behaviour and end up by a cagemate being caved. It is, for example, noteworthy that in the not beak-trimmed tetrads of the first experiment, one individual of rather heavy weight was found in each cage, at the expense of the body-weight of the cage mates (Fig. 4). A similar trend was also found in some cages of NBT triads. Apparently, after some time under these social conditions the cagemates abruptly changed their behaviour, resulting in detrimental effects and great energetic stress in the rest of the group. It might be very interesting to know more about the laying rate, energetics and hormonal state of the energetically dominant *versus* dominated individuals. However, from the corticosterone levels determined no difference was apparent in this chronic situation (see also Cunningham et al., 1988).

There is no doubt that pecking (with a normal beak) at the naked skin of a cagemate, as well as scratching a cagemate's bleeding injuries, cause nociception and, most probably, suffering, i.e. the subjective experience of physiological pain. It can be assumed that such pain caused by conspecifics constitutes a social stress although, strictly speaking, one would require that the behavioural responses observed in harrassed hens are concomitant with reliable indicators of physiological stress, particularly with neuro-hormonal ones. Besides, from the comparisons between different densities in the present experiments, it is not legitimate to conclude that a process of social stress was operative because group-size and floor area/bird happened to be (deliberately) confounded. Had group-size been specifically manipulated independently of floor area, perceptive and/or behavioural adjustments respective to changes in the number of conspecifics would have permitted to interpret the results in terms of social (and not physical) space, and thus possibly also in terms of social stress.

In any event, the present experiments have attempted to devise a *set* of indicators of social stress ascribed to effects of beak-trimming, manipulated as experimental factor in conjunction with cage density. The results showed that these indicators at various levels, some peripheral (e.g. defeathering) and some metabolic (e.g. heat production), proved to be mutually consistent by providing concomitant results. They may in the future prove to constitute relevant and reliable indicators of social stress, in addition to more classical indicators such as adrenocortical responses. Incidentally, it may be recalled that plasma corticosterone levels, assayed at the end of experiment 1 (after 33 weeks) were not affected by the experimental conditions that had induced the very significant differences in defeathering and energetics. Thus, the fact that beak-trimming (in relation to cage density) did clearly affect defeathering, production indices and metabolic rate, would justify to promote the use of a similar set of measures as indicators of social stress in the future, without exclusively focusing on its more traditional hormonal measures. The clear results obtained from the second experiment, which specifically related defeathering with combinations of beak-trimming, support the general hypothesis of an ethologically-induced social stress.

REFERENCES

Adams, A.W., Craig, T.V. and Bhagwat, A.L. 1978. Effects of flock size, age at housing, and mating experience on two strains of egg-type chickens in colony cages. Poult. Sci., 57, 48-53.
Charles, D.R. 1976. The economic importance of feathering. Gleadthorpe Exp. Husb. Farm Poult. Booklet, 25-27.
Clark, J.A., Charles, D.R., Wathes, C.M. and Arrow, J.V. 1975. Heat transfer from haused poultry, its implications for environmental control. World's Poult. Sci. J., 31, 312.
Cunningham, D.L., van Tienhoven, A. and Gvaryahu, G. 1988. Population size, cage area, and dominance rank effects on productivity and well-being of laying hens. Poult. Sci., 67, 399-406.
Doyen, J. and Zayan, R. 1984. Observations on pushing and agression in pairs of hens in battery cages. Behavioural Processes, 9, 171-180.
Geers, R., Michels, H. and Decuypere, E. 1978. Advances in a method for gas analysis in metabolic experiments. Improved calibration of a Noyons diaferometer. Ann. Biol. anim. Bioch. Biophys., 18, 1309-1315.
Herreid, C.F. and Kessel, B.C. 1967. Thermal conductance in birds and mammals. Comp. Biochem. Physiol., 21, 405-414.

Herremans, M. and Decuypere, E. 1986. Heat production of artificially defeathered dwarf cockerels at different ambient temperatures. J. therm. Biol., 11, 127-130.

Herremans, M. and Decuypere, E. 1987. A new approach to recording plumage deterioration. Br. Poult. Sci., 28, 461-470.

Herremans, M. and Decuypere, E. 1988. Interaction of plumage condition and environmental temperature with energetic needs in brown laying hens. Proc. XVIII World's Poultry Congress, Nagoya 1988 : 682-685.

Herremans, M., Decuypere, E., De Groote, G. and De Munter, G. 1988. Invloeden van vedersleet en omgevingstemperatuur op energiebehoeften en produktieparameters bij leghennen. Landbouwtijdschrift, 6, 1387-1404.

Hill, A.T. and Hunt, J.R. 1978. Layer cage depth effects on nervousness, feathering, shell breakage, performance and net egg returns. Poult. Sci., 57, 1204-1216.

Hill, M. 1980. Feather loss in layers. Gleadthorpe Exp. Husb. Farm Poult. Booklet, 7, 46-52.

Hughes, B.O. 1978. The frequency of neck movements in laying hens and the improbability of cage abrasion causing feather wear. Br. Poult. Sci., 19, 289-293.

Hughes, B.O. 1980. Feather damage in hens caged individually. Br. Poult. Sci., 21, 149-154.

Hughes, B.O. 1983. The effects of methionine deficiency and egg production on feather loss in caged layers. Br. Poult. Sci., 24, 549-553.

Hughes, B.O. 1985. Feather loss - how does it occur ? In "Second European symposium on Poultry Welfare" (Ed. R.M. Wegneer). (German Branch of WPSA, Celle) pp. 170-188.

Hughes, B.O. and Duncan, I.J.H. 1972. The influence of strain and environmental factors upon feather pecking and cannibalism. Br. Poult. Sci., 13, 525-547.

Hughes, B.O. and Black, A.J. 1974. The effect of environmental factors on activity, selected behaviour patterns and "fear" of fowls in cages and pens. Br. Poult. Sci., 15, 375-380.

Hughes, B.O. and Black, A.J. 1976. Battery cage shape : its effect on diurnal feeding pattern, egg shell cracking, and feather pecking. Br. Poult. Sci., 17, 327-336.

Hughes, B.O. and Michie, W. 1982. Plumage loss in medium-bodied hybrid hens : the effect of beak trimming and cage design. Br. Poult. Sci. 23, 59-64.

Johnson, R.J., Cumming, R.B. and Farrell, D.J. 1978. The influence of polypeepers and feather-cover on starvation heat production in the laying hen. Aust. J. Agric. Res., 29, 1087-1089.

Kivimaë, A. 1976. The influence of floor area per hen and the number of hens per cage on the performance and behaviour of laying hens. Arch. Geflügelkunde, 40, 202-205.

Koelkebeck, K.W., Amoss, M.S. and Cain, J.R. 1987. Production, physiological, and behavioural responses of laying hens in different management environments. Poult. Sci., 66, 397-407.

Lee, B.D., Morrison, W.D., Leeson, S. and Bayley, M.S. 1983. Effects of feather cover and insulative jackets on metabolic rate of laying hens. Poult. Sci., 62, 1129-1132.

Leeson, S. and Morrison, W.D. 1978. Effect of feather cover on feed efficiency in laying birds. Poult. Sci., 57, 1094-1096.

Li, P.S. and Wagner, W.C. 1983a. Effects of hyperadrenal states on luteinizing hormone in cattle. Biol. of Repr., 29, 11-24

Li, P.S. and Wagner, W.C. 1983b. In vivo and in vitro studies on the effect of adrenocorticotrophic hormone or cortisol on the pituitary response to gonadotrophin releasing hormone. Biol. of Repr., 29, 25-37.

Lucas, A.M. and Stettenheim, P.R. 1972. Avian Anatomy, Integument. Part II. "Agriculture Handbook 362" (U.S. Government Pinting Office, Washington).

Morrison, W.D. and Leeson, S. 1978. Relationship of feed efficiency to carcass composition and metabolic rate in laying birds. Poult. Sci., 57, 735-739.

Nichelmann, M., Oeser, B., Lademann, H. and Grosskopp, C. 1978. Der Einfluss des Befiederungsgrades auf den Wärmehaushalt von Legehennen. In "Die Wirkung von Umweltfactoren auf die Leistungfähigkeit landwirtschaftlicher Nutztiere und ihre Steuerung zur Beeinflussung des Anpassungsvermögens mit dem Ziel der Leistungsbeeinflussung" (Ed. H. Pingel). (Karl-Marx-Universität, Leipzig) pp. 431-440.

O'Neill, S.J.B. and Jackson, N. 1974. Observations on the effect of environmental temperature and environment at moult on the heat production and energy requirements of hens and cockerels of a White Leghorn strain. J. Agric. Sci., 82, 553-558.

Ouart, M. and Adams, A. 1982. Effects of cage design and bird density on layers. 1. Productivity, feathering and nervousness. Poult. Sci., 61, 1606-1613.

Preston, A.P. 1984. Feather pecking in laying cages : Where and When ? Proc. & Abstr. XVII World's Poultry Congr., Helsinki, 433-435.

Ramos, N.C., Anderson, K.E. and Adams, A.W. 1986. Effects of type of cage partition, cage shape and bird density on productivity and well-being of layers. Poult. Sci., 65, 2023-2028.

Richards, S.A. 1977. The influence of loss of plumage on temperature regulation in laying hens. J. Agric. Sci., 89, 393 398.

Romijn, C. 1950. Stofwisselingsonderzoek bij de kip. 2° Mededeling : invloed van verschillende factoren op de calorieproductie. Tijdschrift voor diergeneeskunde, 75, 719-746.

Romijn, C. and Lokhorst, W. 1961. Some aspects of energy metabolism in birds. Proc. 2nd Symp. En. Met., E.A.A.P., 10, 49-59.

Tauson, R. 1980. Cages : how could they be improved ? In "The laying hen and its environment" (Ed. R. Moss) (Martinus Nijhof, Den Haag) pp. 269-304.

Tauson, R. and Svensson, S.A. 1980. Influence of plumage conditions on the hen's feed requirement. Swedish J. Agric. Res., 10, 35-39.

Tullett, S.G., Macleod, M.G. and Jewitt, T.R. 1980. The effects of partial defeathering on energy metabolism in the laying fowl. Br. Poult. Sci., 21, 241-245.

Vanskike, K.P. and Adams, A.W. 1983. Effects of declawing and cage shape on productivity, feathering and fearfulness of egg-type chickens. Poult. Sci., 62, 708.

# PANIC AND HYSTERIA IN DOMESTIC FOWL: A REVIEW.

Andrew D. MILLS and Jean-Michel FAURE

Station de Recherches Avicoles, Institut National de la Recherche Agronomique - Centre de Tours, Nouzilly, 37380 Monnaie, France.

ABSTRACT.

At least in the case of domestic birds, the terms panic and hysteria are used to distinguish outbreaks of hyperexcitability and apparently excessive flight-fright reactions from the behaviour patterns associated with more general flightiness or nervousness. Panic and hysteria are of considerable importance on both economic and welfare grounds and, although hysteria has been most widely documented in flocks of female "layer" type domestic chickens (particularly those of White Leghorn origin), symptoms of panic have been reported in a wide range of breeds and species of domesticated birds.

Although panic and hysteria appear to have many characteristics (hyperexcitability, violent escape reactions and "pile ups" under feeders or against walls) and consequences (physical injuries, suffocation, and drops in production) in common, it is suggested that there are good grounds for believing that they should be considered as distinct phenomena. At least in domesticated birds, panic appears to be expressed only in response to some discernable environmental stimulus or 'trigger' whereas hysteria, which may occur spontaneously and without apparent cause, appears to involve a genotype x environment interaction. Furthermore, outbreaks of hysteria are characterised by events (pre-syndrome shyness, feather pecking, feather eating, increases in food intake and "contagious" waves of excitation or running) which are not usually associated with panic.

The aetiologies of panic and hysteria are complex and appear to have many factors in common. Age, amount of feeding space, availability of nest-boxes, disease, early experience, fear of man or physical injury due to collisions with other birds, nutrition, type or strain of bird, type of husbandry system and, in the case of hysteria, the inappropriate expression of certain social behaviour patterns have all been suggested as potential contributing or causative agents. However, although certain "risk factors" (strain of bird and type of husbandry system) have been identified, no clear cut patterns or chains of causation have been demonstrated for either phenomenon. Various practices and procedures have been suggested as preventative or curative remedies for panic and hysteria. However, many of these involve surgical (debeaking and declawing or amputation of one or more phalanges from each toe) or pharmaceutical (administration of tranquillisers) interventions which are now considered to be unacceptable. Furthermore, all of these methods are effectively "last resorts" and the necessity for their use underlines the lack of knowledge concerning the causations of panic and hysteria. If surgical and pharmaceutical interventions are to be rejected, then, in the absence of a better understanding of the factors leading to panic and hysteria, the occurrence of these phenomena will only be avoided by good husbandry and the use of strains of animals which are not prone to either syndrome.

INTRODUCTION

"Animal experimentation shows that certain combinations of adaptive responses can result in nonadaptive behaviour".

Sidman, (1960).

"Nearly all the behaviour we observe in animals is adaptive. ............................. Animals are certainly not infallible, but when they do make mistakes it is often because they have been transported into an unnatural environment".

Manning, (1979).

These two quotations, although taken from texts not directly related to the behaviour of domesticated birds, illustrate two points directly relevant to the problems of panic and hysteria in domestic fowl, kept under intensive husbandry conditions, which are addressed in this article. Firstly, behaviour patterns which appear to be abnormal to the human observer, may in fact be normal and structured responses in themselves, but inappropriate or redundant in the environment in which the animal finds itself (see also Fox, 1968a; Faure, 1980; Siegel, 1984). Secondly, particular behavioural responses or combinations of such responses, which are adaptive in one environment, may be inadaptive and have deleterious consequences in another.

In domesticated birds, the terms panic and hysteria, have been widely used, not only to describe outbreaks of apparently excessive fright-flight reactions, but also to distinguish such behaviour from the behaviour associated with more general flightiness or nervousness (see; Sanger and Hamdy, 1962; Ferguson,1968; McBride, 1970a; 1970b; Rumsey and Bryan, 1980). However, although, the flight-fright reactions so defined are of considerable importance on both economic and welfare grounds (see Table 1 and below), reference to the literature reveals that, not only have there been few controlled or systematic studies of the aetiologies of panic and hysteria, but also that there is considerable discrepancy between authors in the utilisation and definition of these terms. Therefore, before going into greater detail, it may be of value to consider the common usage meanings of panic and hysteria:

1). Panic; is variously defined as "frantic and sudden fright", or "great terror", without any visible ground or foundation, which is transmissible from one individual to another (MacDonald, 1972; McLeod and Hanks, 1985). In addition, panic is also used, in a modifying sense, to describe "contagious fear responses" which , although they have usually have some discernable cause, are excessive or out of proportion in respect of the stimulus or situation which gives rise to them and may, therefore, have deleterious consequences (McLeod and Hanks, 1984). In animals the term panic has been used in both of these senses. In respect of the first, to describe apparently causeless flight reactions in flocks of 'wild' birds (Campbell and Lack, 1985); in respect of the second, to describe the collective manifestation of unorientated escape behaviour in groups of animals (for example, "stampede" behaviour in turkeys;

[Payne 1959] and frenzied flight behaviour in horses [Schmidt, 1968]).

2). Hysteria, at least in man, is recognised as being a psycho-neurosis, the symptoms of which, although varied and difficult to define exactly ( Campbell, 1977; Lemperière and Féline 1977), include an extreme degree of emotional instability associated with the manifestation of both mental (personality disorders, fits, seizures, etc.) and physical illness (conversion hysteria), (Katz, 1937; MacDonald, 1972; Lemperière and Féline 1977; Campbell, 1977; Delmare and Delmare, 1980). In domesticated birds, the symptoms of hysteria are equally difficult to define but include not only excessive flight fright-flight reaction but also a wide range of other behavioural disorders (see Table 2). In humans, hysteria is believed to stem from some 'internal' (mental) conflict and to have the function of protecting the actor (i.e. the hysterical patient), albeit unknowingly, from some distressing or disturbing situation which he (she) 'cannot deal with' in a more rational manner (Katz, 1937). Within these terms, hysteria is, therefore, a form of irrational or disoriented escape behaviour. However, in the context of this article, it is important to point out that, although Katz (1937) considered hysterical behaviour (in man) to be a regression to a more primitive (sub-human) level of behaviour ("flight from a situation which cannot be met by calm reflection"); the existence of of a true psycho-pathological state of hysteria in animals is debatable (see Katz, 1937; Fox, 1968b; Schmidt, 1968; Lemperière and Féline 1977) and that the use of the term hysteria, in respect of animals, depends largely on the occurrence of what, by subjective comparison with human behaviour, appear to be hysteriform disturbances. Furthermore, although Schmidt (1968) states that "psychic, sensory, motor and autonomic systems are disturbed in ............ hysteria", there is little or no evidence, at least in domestic fowl, that lesions of the central nervous system (Sanger and Hamdy, 1962) or biochemical imbalances are associated with hysteria (Prip, 1976)

TABLE 1.   Economic and welfare related consequences of panic and hysteria in domestic fowl.

| Consequence |
| --- |
| **Lethal** |
| Suffocation (attributable to excessive crowding or pile ups) Disease (egg peritonitis;  caused by secondary infections associated with internal ['intra-uterine'] egg breakage). Trapping and hanging. |
| **Sub-lethal** |
| Bruising (attributable to collisions involved in fright-flight reactions). Increased food intake (associated with feather loss?) Reduced egg output (attributable to internal ['intra-uterine'] breakage and/or breakages associated floor laying). Reduced growth rate (attributable to reduced feed intake associated with hiding?). Skin lesions (attributable to clawing and/or collisions with fixtures and fittings in fright-flight reactions). Feather loss |

At least in animals, panic and hysteria share certain characteristics. Firstly, both involve some form of escape behaviour which is excessive or disorientated and, often, inappropriate to the situation in which it occurs. Secondly, this escape behaviour, because of its excessive or inappropriate nature frequently has deleterious consequences.  In other words a potentially disastrous discrepancy exists between stimulus and response   Perhaps because of this similarity between the symptoms of panic and hysteria, some authors have used the term hysteria, to describe diverse manifestation of escape behaviour in domestic animals (see;  Sanger and Hamdy, 1962;  Chertok and Fontaine, 1963; Fox, 1968b; Keehn, 1979), whereas others have use the term panic to describe, what are essentially, similar behavioural reactions (see Schmidt, 1968). At this point the question arises as to whether or not panic and hysteria are distinct phenomena or merely different manifestations of inappropriate or excessive flight-fright reactions

PANIC AND HYSTERIA IN DOMESTIC BIRDS: DESCRIPTIONS AND DEFINITIONS.

Panic.

In the case of domestic birds, the term panic has been used in at least two senses. These are:

1). Panic running - which is defined as a short period of rapid and unorientated running seen in domestic fowl chicks when placed in a novel environment (such as the open-field - Faure, Jones and Bessei, 1983) or exposed to some unfamiliar auditory or visual stimulus (e.g; eye-like shapes or the ringing of bell - Jones, 1980; Jones and Mills, 1983). This panic running appears to be analogous to the chick's first responses to seek cover when first exposed to danger in the wild and should perhaps be considered to be the normal, if environmentally inappropriate, expression of a fear response (see Archer, 1973; Jones and Faure; 1981a; Faure, Jones and Bessei, 1983; Jones, 1987a).

2). Violent and contagious escape behaviour in 'large' groups of domestic birds - involving wild running, flying and attempts to hide in corners and/or under feeders and drinkers. Such behaviour has been described in broiler fowl, layer fowl, Guinea fowl and turkeys (Golden, 1959; Payne, 1959; Ferguson, 1968; Cauchard, 1971; Anon, 1970 Rhein, 1983). Although sometimes described as being without apparent cause (e.g; Golden, 1959), the expression of panic is usually triggered by some environmental disturbance, which may initially perturb only one animal in a group and then be transmitted (usually very rapidly) to other individuals or affect all individuals in the group more or less simultaneously. This environmental trigger maybe noise (Rhein, 1983), human interventions (Golden, 1959), potential predators or other stimuli which are unfamiliar to the animals (Payne, 1959; Hughes, 1961; Ferguson, 1968; Anon, 1970). Although the exact relationship between fear and panic is uncertain it seems likely that factors which contribute to general fearfulness will also contribute to the expression of panic. Various factors have been suggested as being contributing factors in the expression of fear in both adult birds and chicks ( for reviews, see Duncan, 1985; Jones, 1987a; Jones, 1987b). These include; cage size, cage height (in general birds kept in high level cages tend to be more fearful than birds kept in low level cages - Jones, 1985a), strain and breed of bird (White leghorns and Guinea fowl are notoriously flighty and these same birds appear to be particularly prone to show panic), sex of the birds ( males appear to be less fearful than females in that they respond to environmental disturbance in a more calm or structured way than females - Syme and Syme, 1983; Sefton, 1976; Craig *et al* ,1983), genetic differences within strains or between breeds (Murphy, 1976; Murphy and Wood-Gush, 1978; Faure, 1981a; Craig *et al* , 1983; Jones and Mills, 1983), type of husbandry system and group size (see Syme and Syme, 1983; Hughes and Black, 1974; Craig *et al*., 1983; Duncan, 1985; Jones, 1987a; Jones, 1987b) Of the factors known to influence fear responses, group size appears to be the most important with respect to panic. When birds are kept in large or very large groups (and particularly groups which are of a socially unstructured nature; such as all female 'super' flocks containing several thousand birds of identical ages) mechanisms for the regulation of fear responses appear to breakdown (Hughes, 1982) and panic results as a consequence of a form of positive feedback mechanism, in which fear is transmitted from one bird to another in an ever increasing fashion.  In this sense, panic would appear to be a reflexively socially facilitated behaviour pattern (see Clayton, 1978).  In small groups of birds, where social relationships and social structure are well defined, this positive feedback does not appear to occur and activity (fear responses) caused by some disturbing event quickly die away as a result of habituation (Hughes, 1982) or, perhaps, as is the case with aggression, the presence of dominant birds in all female groups (Craig *et al* ,1969; Ylander and Craig, 1980) or males in mixed flocks (Craig and Bhagwat, 1974) inhibits violent behavioural reactions in lower ranking birds.  There is little evidence available concerning the group sizes at which this breakdown in the control of fear responses will occur and it seem likely that this will vary with species, strain and flock structure. However, Craig and Adams (1984) point out that that the incidences of panic and hysteriform behaviour increase rapidly when group size exceeds twelve

A tentative definition of panic, at least in domestic fowl, might therefore be;  'the excessive and inappropriate expression of reflexive socially facilitated fear (flight-fright) responses attributable to breakdowns in the normal control of social behaviour.which occur when birds are kept in large socially unstructured groups'.

## Hysteria.

Hysteria, or hysteriform behaviour, in groups chickens was first reported in the late 1950's and early 1960's and was initially described as "a strange fright-flight behaviour" (Sanger and Hamdy, 1962), characterised by the expression of extreme nervousness followed, firstly, by squawking and flight for no apparent reason and then by hiding or crowding in corners or under feeders and waterers.  Peculiar characteristics of these outbreaks were that they tended to be repeated at regular intervals (approximately every 5 to 10 minutes in the first reports), involved only females and affected the various birds in a group in a 'progressive' fashion (that is to say, 'waves of excitement or running behaviour would 'sweep' through a flock but not affect all members of the group simultaneously). Although the most obvious symptoms of avian hysteria, like panic, were disorientated flight-fright reactions (involving birds running or flying into one another, into stockmen and into fixtures and fittings), a distinction was been made between the two traits, not only because hysteria had the peculiar characteristics mentioned above, but also because outbreaks of hysteria were generally accompanied by a variety of behavioural vices or anomalies which were not invariably associated with outbreaks of panic (see Table 2).

Because of the very severe economic consequences of outbreaks of hysterifom behaviour ( in particular, substantial mortality and reduced egg production - Sanger and Hamdy, 1962), the syndrome has attracted considerable attention, particularly in the popular poultry press, but even to date there have been few systematic studies of its causation. This deficit undoubtedly stems from the fact that outbreaks of hysteria are sporadic and difficult to induce experimentally (see Ruszler and Quisenberry [1979] for a specific example concerning the effects of declawing on hysteria and Faure [1981b] for a general discussion of the problems associated with studies of non-inducible behaviour). A wide range of behavioural, environmental, nutritional and miscellaneous factors have been suggested as causal or contributing factors in outbreaks of hysteria ( see Table 3). However, few of these have been demonstrated consistently and the causation of hysteria obviously requires further discussion. Setting aside the facts that reference to the literature indicates that outbreaks of hysteria are almost exclusively confined to large groups of female layer type birds of White Leghorn origin (two reports of hysteria in broiler type fowl of unspecified genetic origin also exist - Sanger and Hamdy, 1962), the factors which have been most dogmatically suggested as causal factors for hysteria are feather pecking and cannibalism (Rumsey and Bryan, 1980), pain associated with clawing injuries (Hansen, 1970), nutritional deficiencies - in particular vitamin B deficiencies (see Table 3 for references) and the abnormal expression of flock formation behaviour (McBride, 1970a; 1970b).

TABLE 2. Factors implicated in or associated with outbreaks of hysteria as distinct from panic.

| Factor | Reference |
| --- | --- |
| Cannibalism. | Hansen, 1969; Prip, 1975; 1976; 1977. |
| Feather pecking (auto or self pecking). | Sanger & Hamdy, 1962. |
| Feather pecking (directed at other birds) | Jamieson, 1964; Jackson, 1970; Prip, 1975; 1976; 1977; Rumsey & Bryan, 1980. |
| Feather eating. | Sanger & Hamdy, 1962; Rumsey & Bryan, 1980. |
| Feather loss. | Prip, 1975; 1976; 1977; Rott, 1978; Rumsey & Bryan, 1980. |
| Increased food intake. | Sanger & Hamdy, 1962. |
| Pre-outbreak shyness or nervousness | Sanger & Hamdy, 1962; Prip, 1975; 1976; 1977; Rumsey & Bryan, 1980. |
| Reduced food intake. | Hughes, 1961 |
| Sex of birds (only females affected). | Sanger & Hamdy, 1962; McBride, 1970a; 1970b; Prip, 1975; 1976; 1977.. |
| Strain of bird (predominately White Leghorns). | Ferguson, 1968; Prip, 1975; 1976; 1977 |

Although, feather pecking and cannibalism are frequently associated with outbreaks of hysteria, evidence for their playing a key role in the causation of hysteria is scanty. Feather pecking and cannibalism do not appear to be present in all flocks which present hysteriform behaviour and standard measures for the prevention of feather pecking and cannibalism are not necessarily effective in preventing hysteria (see Table 4). The simultaneous occurrence of feather pecking, cannibalism and hysteria is more likely to be a consequence of generally poor environmental conditions than it is evidence for a causal link between the three traits. The role of pain attributable to clawing injuries in the causation of hysteria seems equally uncertain. Although declawing (amputation of one or more phalanges from each toe) has consistently been claimed to be effective in preventing hysteria (see Table 4) and claw trimming to be effective just until the claws regrow; the only systematic study of the effects of declawing by Ruzler and Quinsenberry (1979) was inconclusive, since hysteria did not appear in the treated or control animals, despite these authors attempts to provoke its expression. Furthermore, the argument that hysteriform behaviour leads to clawing injuries and that clawing leads to hysteria seems to be somewhat circular, although the possibility of clawing originally arising as a consequence of some other behaviour such as panic cannot be ignored. Evidence concerning the role of nutritional factors in hysteria is confusing. Various authors have reported successfully treating or preventing outbreaks of hysteria with various dietary supplements, whereas others have found the same or essentially similar treatments to be without effect (see Table 4), this situation being further complicated by differences in experimental procedures or conditions and, in some cases, the absence of any form of control. For example, vitamin B deficiency has been suggested as a cause of hysteria in caged birds which cannot ingest droppings and thereby obtain a supplement of microbially formed vitamin (see Prip, 1975). Yet birds kept on the floor also show hysteria, blood levels of vitamin B are similar in affected and unaffected birds (Prip, 1975) and niacin supplements are not invariably successful in suppressing or preventing hysteria (Table 4). Finally, McBride's (1970a; 1970b) hypothesis that hysteria is the inappropriate expression of a brood dispersal and flock formation behaviour pattern, known as "streaming", does not appear to be consistent with many descriptions of the conditions associated with outbreaks of hysteria. Streaming occurs in feral populations of birds at or about the time of sexual maturity. During streaming young males begin to run short distances away from their natal group followed by females from their own and nearby groups, this procedure being repeated several times until broods have been broken up and mixed in to new independent flocks. However, if hysteria is the inappropriate expression of streaming behaviour, then hysteria should only occur in birds at about the age of sexual maturity, infact hysteria has been reported in birds as young as seven to eight weeks of age (Hansen, 1970; Chawla *et al*, 1973) and as old as to fifty two weeks of age (Reynolds and Maplesden, 1977)..

It would therefore appear that there is no clear cut cause of hysteria and reference to Table 3 shows that almost any form of environmental abuse or adversity is likely to contribute to outbreaks of hysteria. However, amongst these contributing factors strain of bird (White Leghorn), group size (which implicitly includes type of husbandry system) and flock structure (in that they are the most consistently cited contributing factors) appear to be the most important. At this point it becomes possible to suggest that outbreaks of hysteria are not attributable to any one particular causal factor but rather to a complex genotype x environment reaction which more likely than not involves a threshold effect (see also Rott, 1978). That is to say if birds of hysteria 'prone' strain are kept in large unstructured flocks and then subjected to a further range of adversive factors, these additional adversive factors act in an additive fashion and their cumulative effects 'push' the birds beyond a hypothetical threshold for the expression of hysteriform behaviour (for a fuller description of the principles underlying threshold effects in general, see; Wright [1934] and Fuller and Thompson [1960]). It is pertinent to point out here that Hughes (1961) has also suggested that threshold effects may be implicated in the expression of hysteria, although his model implicates only interactions between environmental and nutritional factors and rejects a role for genetic factors. A genotype x environment threshold effect model of the expression of hysteria explains not only the predisposition of White Leghorns to show hysteriform behaviour (such birds are genetically close to the threshold) but also the diversity and sometimes apparently contradictory nature of the various behavioural, environmental, nutritional and miscellaneous factors which have been associated with outbreaks of hysteria. In this last context, the important point about such a threshold model is that any combination of adversive factors may act to 'push' the birds beyond the point at which hysteriform behaviour is likely to occur; i.e. it is not the exact nature of the stimuli involved that matters only their cumulative effects.

A tentative definition of hysteria might therefore be 'a syndrome of behavioural vices (cannibalism, feather pecking, feather eating, nervousness and excessive flight fright reactions with or without apparent cause) which is associated with keeping female birds of similar ages in large flocks and is triggered when a complex additive interaction between genotype and environment exceeds a threshold point'.

TABLE 3. Factors implicated in or associated with outbreaks of hysteria

| Factor | Reference |
| --- | --- |
| Behavioural. | |
| Abnormal expression of flock formation behaviour. | McBride, 1970a; 1970b |
| Cannibalism and feather pecking. | Rumsey and Bryan, 1980 |
| Environmental. | |
| Management failures (Food and water deprivation). | Prip, 1975; 1976; 1977. |
| Poor ventilation (high dust and ammonia levels. | Prip, 1975; 1976; 1977; Rumsey & Bryan,1980. |
| Excessive or unfamiliar noise. | Prip, 1975; 1976; 1977. |
| Electro-shockers on feeders. | Prip, 1975; 1976; 1977; Rumsey & Bryan,1980. |
| Low temperature. | Rott, 1978. |
| Increases in temperature. | Sanger & Hamdy, 1962. |
| High stocking densities and large flock sizes. | Sanger & Hamdy, 1962; Elmslie et al.,1966; Hansen, 1969; 1970; Rott, 1978; Halik et al.,1979; Craig et al., 1983. |
| Type of husbandry system (collective cages and large floor houses). | Elmslie et al., 1966; Hansen, 1976; Prip, 1975; 1976; 1977; Rumsey & Bryan, 1980. |
| Inadequate feeding space. | Prip, 1975; 1976; 1977. |
| Contact with humans (husbandry procedures, vaccinations etc.). | Sanger & Hamdy, 1962; Jamieson, 1964. |
| Nutritional deficiencies. | |
| Magnesium and calcium | Prip, 1975; 1976; 1977. |
| Vitamin B | Prip, 1975; 1976; 1977. |
| Sulphur amino acids | Prip, 1975; 1976; 1977. |

. TABLE 3 (continued). Factors implicated in or associated with out breaks of hysteria.

| Factor | Reference |
|---|---|
| Miscellaneous | |
| Disease (especially of the G.I. tract). | Rumsey & Bryan, 1980. |
| Pain (associated with injuries due to clawing in flight reactions). | Hansen, 1970. |
| Age of birds | Jamieson, 1964; McBride, 1970a; 1970b; Prip, 1975; 1976; 1977; Reynolds & Maplesden, 1977. |
| Sex of birds (only females affected). | Sanger & Hamdy, 1962; McBride, 1970a; 1970b; Prip, 1975; 1976; 1977. |
| Strain of bird (predominately White Leghorns). | Ferguson, 1968; Prip, 1975; 1976; 1977. |

PREVENTION AND TREATMENT OF PANIC AND HYSTERIA.

Although limiting group size and, where possible, avoiding flighty strains of birds would appear to be obvious methods for reducing the incidence of outbreaks of panic, there appear to be few other solutions presently available other than attempting to limit the occurrence of situations or stimuli which might trigger outbreaks or trying to 'calm' birds at critical times during husbandry. For examples, reduced lighting (Golden, 1959) and tranquilizers (Champion *et al.*, 1966; Parker, 1969) have been suggested as methods for reducing flight-fright reactions in broiler fowl at time of capture for slaughter. Other methods for reducing the incidence of panic appear, at least at present, to be either untested under commercial conditions or only in the early stages of development. However, such methods include, the development of new automated husbandry techniques which reduce the adversive nature of certain traditional techniques (for example, the use of automatic harvesting machines for the capture of broiler fowl which appears to induce less fear in the birds than does manual capture – Duncan *et al*, 1986) and attempting to increase the thresholds for the release of fear behaviour either by ontogenetic (such as handling during early life – Jones and Faure, 1981b) or genetic (Faure,1979; Jones, 1985b) means.

A wide variety of treatments for hysteria have been attempted but have had very mixed success (Table 3). This situation undoubtedly reflects the complicated causation of hysteria, in that the balance of factors contributing to outbreaks of hysteriform behaviour probably differs between flocks and thus treatments which are effective in one flock may be ineffective in another. Furthermore, the extent to which surgical interventions (such as beak trimming or declawing) and the use of tranquilizers will be effective in preventing or suppressing outbreaks of hysteria is open to question. Certainly, if feather pecking, cannibalism and pain due to clawing injuries are likely to be major contributing factors to outbreaks of hysteria, then beak trimming and declawing are likely to be of some value, but questions remain outstanding as to the acceptability of such practices as standard husbandry procedures. The use of sedatives or tranquilizers appears to hold little promise for the treatment or prevention of hysteria for the following reasons: Firstly, at least in laying hens they do not appear to be particularly effective either as curative (see Table 3 for references) or preventative measures (Hansen, 1972). Secondly, they are expensive (Faure, 1979), and, thirdly, they pose problems of residues (again particularly in the case of laying hens – Reynolds and Maplesden, 1977; Faure, 1979). Thus, although certain miscellaneous treatments such as the play back to affected flocks of recordings of male crows or sounds from unaffected flocks has been reported to have beneficial effects in some cases (Jamieson, 1964; Chawla *et al*.,1973; Hughes, 1961; Jackson, 1970), it seems likely that hysteria can only be prevented by judicious choice of the strain of birds used, keeping group size to the minimum possible and ensuring that all aspects of husbandry are carefully controlled at all times.

TABLE 4. Preventative and curative treatments for hysteria

| Treatment | Effective* | Reference |
|---|---|---|
| **Environmental** | | |
| Reduced lighting | No | Sanger & Hamdy, 1962; Prip, 1976. |
| Red lighting | No | Hansen, 1969; 1970; Prip, 1975; 1976; 1977. |
| Blue lighting | No | Hansen, 1970. |
| Blue then white lighting. | No | Hansen, 1970. |
| Reduce temperature (down to 0°C) | No | Sanger & Hamdy, 1962. |
| Constant temperature (22.2 °C). | Yes | Rumsey & Bryan, 1980. |
| Increase temperature | No | Prip,1975; 1976; 1977. |
| Increased ventilation | Yes | Rumsey & Bryan, 1980. |
| Reducing flock size | Yes | Sanger & Hamdy, 1962 Elmslie *et al*., 1966. |
| | No | Sanger & Hamdy, 1962 |
| Mixing affected and unaffected flocks | Yes | Hughes, 1961; Sanger & Hamdy, 1962; Chawla *et al*., 1973. |
| Transferring affected birds from the floor to cages. | Yes | Jamieson, 1964. |
| **Nutritional** | | |
| High roughage feeds. | No | Sanger & Hamdy, 1962 |

TABLE 4 (continued). Preventative and curative treatments for hysteria.

| Treatment | Effective* | Reference |
|---|---|---|
| **Nutritional (continued).** | | |
| High protein diet. | Yes. | Rumsey & Bryan,1980. |
| | No | Sanger & Hamdy, 1962; Prip, 1975; 1976; 1977. |
| Niacin supplement | Yes. | Schutz, 1965; Hansen, 1969; Petersen, 1972. |
| | No | Hansen,1972;1976; Chawla *et al*.,1973; Prip, 1975; 1976. 1977. |
| Cysteine + Lysine + + methionine supplement. | Yes | Rumsey & Bryan, 1980. |
| Thiamine supplement | No | Prip, 1976. |
| NaCl supplement. | No | Prip, 1976 |
| **Surgical interventions** | | |
| Beak trimming | Yes | Hughes, 1961; Jamieson, 1964 Rumsey & Bryan, 1980. |
| Beak trimming | No | Chawla *et al*., 1973. |
| Claw trimming. | Yes | Hansen, 1969; 1970. |
| De-clawing. | Yes | Hughes, 1961; Hansen, 1970; 1972; Ruzler & Quinsberry, 1979. |
| **Drug therapy** | | |
| Furazolide | No | Sanger & Hamdy, 1962; |
| Chloropromazine | No | Chawla et al., 1973. |
| Reserpine (various forms,doses and methods | Yes | Hughes,1961; Reynolds & Maplesden, 1977. |
| of administration) | No | Sanger & Hamdy, 1962; Hansen, 1970; 1976. |
| Unspecified sedatives | No | Prip, 1976 |

TABLE 4 (continued). Preventative and curative treatments for hysteria.

| Treatment | Effective* | Reference |
|---|---|---|
| Miscellaneous | | |
| Spraying birds with cold water. | No | Sanger & Hamdy, 1962. |
| Playing radio music | No | Sanger & Hamdy, 1962; Prip, 1976. |
| Play back of vocalisations from flocks of unaffected birds. | Yes | Hughes, 1961; Jackson, 1970. |
| Presence of males in flock | Yes | Jamieson, 1964; Chawla *et al.* 1973.. |
| | No. | Prip, 1976. |

*In this table the terms Yes and No are not used definitively but rather in the qualified sense of describing generally positive or negative reports of the effects of a given treatment or treatments.

GENERAL DISCUSSION AND CONCLUSIONS.

The Introduction of this paper commenced with two quotations. The first of these, from Sidman (1960), emphasizes the fact that under certain conditions behaviour which is normally adaptive may become inadaptive. The second, from Manning (1979) draws attention to the role of environmental factors in the appearance of abnormal behaviour patterns. Panic, which was defined here as the "excessive and inappropriate expression of reflexive socially facilitated fear (flight-fright) responses" would appear to fall into the category of behaviour patterns envisaged by Sidman. The function of fear behaviour is to protect the actor from some actual or potential source of danger (Salzen, 1979; Jones, 1987a). However, when fear responses develop into panic their adaptive value is lost and the behaviour becomes inadaptive in that it has no protective function and may directly or indirectly (because of the environment in which the animal is kept) lead to injuries and stress (Jones,1985b). The manifestation of the diverse syndrome of abnormal behaviour patterns associated with avian hysteria would, on the other hand, appear to be a reflection of an interaction between genotype and environment in the sense envisaged in the quotation from Manning. The diverse and sometimes contradictory list of factors which have (or have not) been implicated in outbreaks of hysteria would appear to support this view Reference to Table 3 shows that virtually any form of environmental abuse or mishap is likely to contribute to outbreaks of hysteriform behaviour and that female birds of White Leghorn origin are particularly prone to the expression of such behaviour. Such an aetiology is difficult to explain except in terms of the polygenic threshold model proposed above and it would therefore appear that avian hysteria is, in itself, not a specific response but rather a generalized (if extreme) response to environmental adversities. With the argument couched in such terms it becomes clear that panic and hysteria in domesticated birds are distinct phenomena. However, it is important to point out here that both traits share causal factors and both are chartacterised by apparently excessive flight fright reactions. Indeed, it is possible to argue that the occurrence of panic will contribute to the probability of hysteria occurring. Given this, and the facts that genotype and group size appear to be the major contributing factors for both traits, the judicious choice of animals and limiting group size (which would probably have additional benefits with respect to welfare – Hughes, 1988) combined with the careful control of environmental conditions would go some way to reducing, if not eliminating both panic and hysteria.

REFERENCES.

Anonymous, 1970. Clipping turkey toes to reduce down-grading. Poultry Digest, 29; 171.

Archer, J. 1973. Effects of testosterone on tonic immobility responses in the young male chick. 1970. Behav. Biol., 8; 551 - 556.

Campbell, B. and Lack, E. (Eds.) 1985. A dictionary of birds. (The British Ornithologist's Union; T and A.D. Poyser Ltd, Calton).

Campbell, R 1977. Le comportement humain - Lé déséquillibre mental. (Time-Life International [Nederland] B.V.)

Champion, L.R., Zindel, H.C., Ringer, R.K. and Wolford, H.H. 1966. The performance of starter pullets treated with SU-9064 (Pacitran) prior to transport. Poultry Sci., 45; 1359 - 1368.

Cauchard, J.C. 1971. La pintade (*Numida meleagris*). (Editions Henri Peladan; Uzés [Gard])

Chawla, R.S., Singh, B. and Grewal, G.S. 1973. Avian hysteria - preliminary observations. Gujvet, 7: 74 - 76.

Chertok, L. and Fontaine, M. 1963. Psychosomatics in veterinary medicine. J. Psychosomatic Res., 7: 229 - 235.

Clayton, D.A. 1978. Socially facilitated behaviour. Q. Rev. Biol., 53; 373 - 392.

Craig, J.V. and Adams, A.W. 1984. Behaviour and well-being of hens (*Gallus Domesticus*) in alternative housing environments. Wld's Poultry Sci. J. 40; 221 - 240.

Craig, J.V. and Bhagwat, A.L. 1974. Agonistic and mating behaviour of adult chickens modified by social and physical environments. Appl. Anim. Ethol., 1; 57 - 65.

Craig, J.V., Biswas, D.K. and Guhl, A.M. 1969. Agonistic behaviour influenced by strangeness, crowding and heredity in female domestic fowl. Anim. Behav., 17; 498 - 506.

Craig, J.V., Craig, T.P. and Dayton, A.D. 1983. Fearful behaviour by hens of two genetic stocks. Appl. Anim. Ethol., 10; 263 - 273.

Delamare, J. and Delmare, J. 1980. Dictionnaire des termes techniques de medecine (20th edition). (Maloine S.A.; Paris).

Duncan, I.J.H. 1985. How do fearful birds respond, In: Proc. 2nd European symposium on poultry welfare. (Ed. R. Wegner; German branch of the W.P.S.A). pp. 95 - 106.

Duncan, I.J.H., Slee, G.S., Kettlewell, P., Berry, P. and Carlisle, A.J. 1986. Comparison of the stressfulness of harvesting broiler chickens by machine and by hand. Brit. Poultry Sci. 27; 109 - 114.

Elmslie, L.J., Jones, R.H. and Knight, D.W. 1966. A general theory describing the effects of varying flock size and stocking density on the performance of caged layers. In: Proc. 13th World's Poultry Congress. (Eds. E.A. Dunyunov, G. Kopylovskaya, G.K. Penionzhkevich, E.E., N.V. Pigarev and A.P. Valdman; Kiev, U.S.S.R.). pp. 490 - 495.

Faure, J.M. 1979. Sélection génétique et stress. Proc. Conf. le 10 mai 1979 à Tours lors d'un seminaire GTV-INRA. pp. 53 - 59.

Faure, J.M. 1980. To adapt the bird to the environment or the bird to the environment. In: The laying hen and its environment. (Ed. R. Moss). Current topics in veterinary medicine and animal science. Volume 8. (Martinus Nijhoff Publishers; The Hague). pp. 19 - 30.

Faure, J.M. 1981a. Analyse génétique de l'activité précoce en open-field du jeune poussin (Gallus gallus domesticus). These d'Etat, Faculté des Sciences, Univ. de Toulouse, N°. d'ordre 1010. 345 pp.

Faure, J.M. 1981b. Behavioural measures for selection. In: Report of Proc. 1st European symposium on Poultry welfare. (Ed. L.Y. Sørensen; Danish Branch of the W.P.S.A.). pp. 35 - 41.

Faure, J.M., Jones, R.B. and Bessei, W. 1983. Fear and social motivation as factors in the open-field behaviour of the domestic chick. A theoretical consideration. Biol. Behav., 8; 103 - 116.

Ferguson, W. 1968. Abnormal behaviour in domestic birds. In: Abnormal behaviour in animals. (Ed. M.W. Fox). (W.B. Saunders Company), Philadelphia; London, Toronto). pp. 188 - 207.

Fox, M.W. 1968a. Introduction: The concepts of normal and abnormal behaviour. In: Abnormal behaviour in animals. (Ed. M.W Fox). (W.B. Saunders Company; Philadelphia, London, Toronto). pp. 1 - 5.

Fox, M.W. 1968b. Psychomotor disturbances. In: Abnormal behaviour in animals. (Ed. M.W. Fox). (W.B. Saunders Company; Philadelphia, London, Toronto). pp. 356 - 364.

Fuller, J.L. and Thompson, R.T. 1960. Behaviour genetics (John Wiley and Sons Inc.; New York, London).

Golden, E.F. 1959 Broilers: Production and management (2nd edition), (Poultry World; London).

Halik, J., Zavodsky, I. and Sestak, K. 1979. Hysteria of fowl. Veterinarstvi, 29; 361 - 362.

Hansen, R.S. 1969. Removal of toenails stopped hysteria. Poultry Digest, 28: 457.

Hansen, R.S. 1970. Hysteria of mature hens in cages. Poultry Sci., 49: 1392 - 1393.

Hansen, R.S. 1972. Influence of several treatments on hysteria of mature hens. Poultry Sci. 51: 1814 - 1815.

Hansen, R.S. 1976. Nervousness and hysteria of mature female chickens. Poultry Sci., 55: 531 - 543.

Hughes, B.O. 1982. The social behaviour of the fowl. Appl. Anim. Ethol., 9; 84 - 85.

Hughes, B.O. 1988. Current knowledge of bird welfare requirements. Wld's Poultry Sci. J., 44; 62 - 63.

Hughes, B.O. and Black, A.J. 1974. The effects of environmental factors on activity, selected behaviour patterns and "fear of fowls in cages and pens. Brit. Poultry Sci., 15; 375 - 380.

Hughes, W.F. 1961. Preliminary observations on avian hysteria. Avian Dis., 5; 351 -352.

Jackson, D. 1970. Sound therapy for avian hysteria. Poultry Digest, 290; 286 - 287.

Jamieson, S.L. 1964. Some observations on hysteria in chickens. Pacific Poultryman (Poultry Tribune), 70; 20 - 48.

Jones, R.B; 1980. Reactions of male domestic chicks to two-dimensional eye-like shapes. Anim. Behav., 28; 212 - 218

Jones, R.B. 1985a. Fearfulness of hens caged individually or in groups in different tiers of a battery and the effects of translocation between tiers. Brit. Poultry Sci., 26; 399 - 408.

Jones, R.B. 1985b. Fearfulness and adaptability in the domestic fowl. IRCS Med. Sci. 13; 797 - 800.

Jones, R.B. 1987a. The assessment of fear in the domestic fowl. In: Cognitive aspects of social behaviour in the domestic fowl. (Eds. R. Zayan and I.J.H. Duncan), (Elsevier; Amsterdam, Oxford, New york, Tokyo). pp. 40 - 81.

Jones, R.B. 1987b. Social aspects of fear in the domestic fowl. In: Cognitive aspects of social behaviour in the domestic fowl. (Eds. R. Zayan and I.J.H. Duncan), (Elsevier; Amsterdam, Oxford, New york, Tokyo). pp. 82 - 149.

Jones, R.B. and Faure, J.M. 1981a. Open-field behaviour of male and female domestic chicks as a function of housing conditions and novelty. Biol. Behav., 7; 17 - 25.

Jones, R.B. and Faure, J.M. 1981b The effects of regular handling on fear responses in the domestic chick. Biol. Behav., 6; 135 - 143.

Jones, R.B and Mills, A.D., 1983. Estimation of fear in two lines of domestic chicks: correlations between various methods and measures. Behav. Processes, 8; 243 - 253.

Katz, D. 1937. Animals and man. (Penguin books; Melbourne, London, Baltimore).

Keehn, J.D. 1979. Psychopathology in animal and man. In: Psychopathology in animals. (Ed. J.D. Keehn; Academic Press Inc.; New York). pp. 1 - 27.

Lemperiére, T. and Feline, A. 1977. Abrégé de psychiatrie de l'adulte. (Masson; Paris, New York, Barcelona, Milan).

MacDonald, A.M. (Ed.), 1972. 'Chambers' 20th century dictionary. (W & R

Chambers Ltd; Edinburgh).

McBride, G. 1970a. The social control of behaviour in fowls. In: Aspects of poultry behaviour. (Eds. B.M. Freeman and R.F. Gordon), (British Poultry Science; Edinburgh). pp. 3 - 13.

McBride, G. 1970b. Understanding the hen. Poultry Digest, 29; 16 - 19.

McLeod, W.T. and Hanks, P. (Eds) 1985. The new 'Collins' concise dictionary of the English language. (W.M. Collins Sons & Co. Ltd; London).

Manning, A. 1979. An introduction to animal behaviour. Third edition. (Edward Arnold [Publishers] Limited; London).

Murphy, L.B. 1976. A study of of behavioural expression of fear and exploration in in two stocks of domestic fowl. Ph.D. Thesis, Univ. of Edinburgh, 343 pp.

Murphy, L.B. and Wood-Gush, D.G.M., 1978. The interpretation of the behaviour of domestic fowl in strange environments. Biol. Behav., 3; 39 - 61.

Parker, E.L. 1969. Metoserpate hydrochloride - tranquilizer for specific stresses in poultry. Feedstuffs 11; 21 - 22.

Payne, L.F 1959. Turkeys grown in confinement and on the range. Poultry Sci. 38; 1087 - 1094.

Petersen, E.H., 1972. Serviceman's poultry health handbook (2nd printing), (Better Poultry Health Company; Pavetteville, Arkansas, U.S.A.).

Prip, M., 1975. Hysteria in laying hens. Wld's Poultry Sci. J., 31; 306 - 308.

Prip, M., 1976. Hysteria in laying hens. In: Proc. 5th European Poultry Conference. Vol. 2. (World's Poultry Science Association [Malta branch]). pp. 1062 - 1069.

Prip, M., 1977. Hysteria in laying hens. Poultry International (October, 1977); 10 - 18.

Reynolds, W.A. and Maplesden, D.C. 1977. Monoserpate hydrochloride for the treatment of hysteria in replacement pullets. Avian Dis., 21; 720 - 725.

Rhein, B. 1983. Effect of aircraft noise on mortality and productivity of broilers and hens. Unpublished Inaugural dissertation. (Tierarztliche Hochscule; Hanover). pp. 1 - 90.

Rott, M., 1978. Behavioural disorder in intensively kept poultry - cause and importance of hysteria. Monatshefte fur Veterinarmedizin, 33; 455 - 458.

Rumsey, R.R. and Bryan, T. 1980. Hysteria in laying flocks. Poultry Digest: 39; 37 - 38.

Ruszler, P.L. and Quisenberry, J.H. 1979. The effects of declawing two flock sizes of 23-week-old pullets on hysteria and certain production traits. Poultry Sci., 58; 778 - 784.

Salzen, E.A. 1979. The ontogeny of fear in animals. In: Fear in animals and man. (Ed. W. Sluckin). (Van Nostrand Rheinhold, Co.; New York). pp. 125 -

163.

Sanger, V.L. and Hamdy, A.H. 1962. A strange fright/flight behaviour pattern (hysteria) in hens. J. Amer. Vet. Assoc., 140: 455 - 459.

Schutz, J.V. 1965. Feeding niacin controls hysteria. Poultry Digest, 24: 179.

Schmidt, J.P. 1968. Psychosomatics in veterinary medicine. In: Abnormal behaviour in animals. (Ed. M.W. Fox). (W.B. Saunders Company; Philadelphia, London,Toronto). pp. 356 - 364.

Sefton, A.E. 1976. The interaction of cage size, cage level, social density , fearfulness and production of single comb White leghorns. Poultry Sci., 55: 1922 - 1926.

Sidman, M. 1960. Normal sources of pathological behaviour. Science, 132: 61 - 68.

Siegel, P.B. 1984. The role of behaviour in poultry production: A review of research. Appl. Anim. Ethol., 11: 299 - 316.

Syme, L.A. and Syme, G.J. 1983. Position in the peck order and response to human threat in domestic fowl. Appl. Anim. Ethol., 9; 351 - 357.

Wright, S. 1934. The results of crosses between inbred strains of guinea pigs differing in numbers of digits. Genetics, 19: 537 - 551.

Ylander, D.M. and Craig, J.V. 1980. Inhibition of agonistic acts between domestic hens by a dominant third party. Appl. Anim. Ethol., 6; 63 - 69.

SESSION V : CONTROL OF SOCIAL STRESS

CONTROL OF SOCIAL STRESS BY CONSIDERATION OF SUITABLE SOCIAL SPACE

K. Zeeb, Ch. Bock, B. Heinzler
Institute of Animal Hygiene
7800 Freiburg, Bundesrepublik Deutschland

ABSTRACT

We proceed at the consumption that a certain degree of locomotion is an expression of social stress in cattle. Cows in
cubicle houses need a walking space of at least 3,5 m²/cow.
More walking space per cow reduces stress and as a result of
this locomotion. Inferior cows suffer from stress if in the
cow house there is not at least one feeding place per cow available. The qualification of the herdsman's ability to keep cattle
has an influence on the social stress of cattle. Low qualification of the herdsman produces social stress and therefore more
locomotor activity.

Social stress in cattle is to be reduced by consideration
of sufficient walking space, feeding place, number of cubicles
and the improvement of the herdsman's qualification to keep
cattle.

WALKING SPACE AND LOCOMOTOR ACTIVITY

Cows need a walking space of at least 3,5 m²/600 kg body-
weight. (Fig. 1).

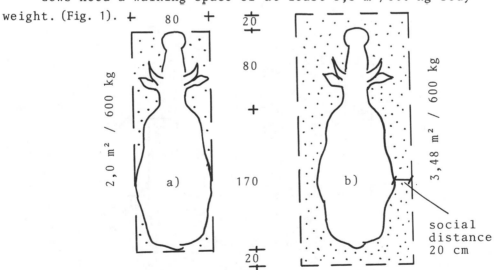

Fig. 1   Dimension of the walking space/Cow
         a) agreeing only to the measurements of body
         b) including the social distance.

There is a decreasing tendency when comparing the locomotion of cows in different cubicle housing units of different walking space per animal: < 3,0; 3,0 - 4,0;> 4,0 m² (Fig. 2). The difference of locomotion is caused by the decreasing of the social pressure which is induced by the increasing walking space. For inferior cows food competition means social stress. We found a high significant correlation between social competition and locomotor activity: $r_s$ = -0,842 (p<0,01), n = 10 farms. Furthermore we found that the difference of numbers of injuries between dominant and inferior cows was significant:  p <0,05; n = 100 animals.

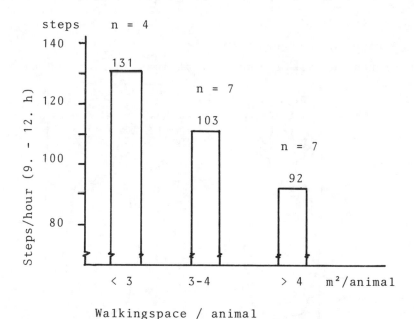

Fig. 2  Walkingspace and steps/hour

## NUMBER OF FEEDING PLACES AND DISPLACEMENTS

Fig. 3 shows that in 12 farms with a feeding place/animal relation of <1:1 there were less displacements in the feeding area than in 18 farms with a relation of >1:1; there was a difference of 22 %. We found a low negativ significant correlation between social competition and numbers of feeding places :
$r_s$ = -0,568 (p <0,1), n = 11 farms.

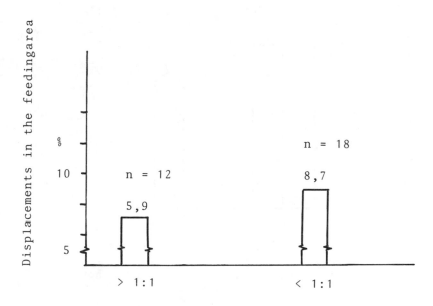

Fig. 3   Displacements in the feeding area
         during the first hour after serving feed

## NUMBERS OF CUBICLES AND LOCOMOTOR ACTIVITY

If there is not one cubicle for each cow available social stress for inferior cows will be the result. In 8 farms with a cubicle/cow relation  of < 1:1 more locomotion did occur in the first hours past midnight than in 10 farms with a relation of >1:1(Fig. 4); there was a difference of 23 %.

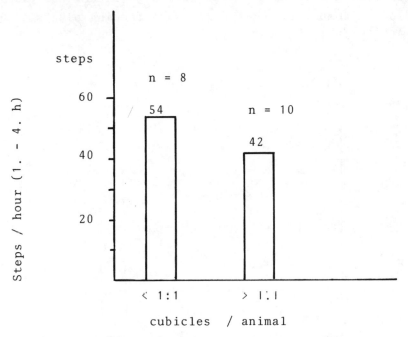

Fig. 4    Cubicles  /animal  and steps / hour

## THE HERDSMAN'S QUALIFICATION

Insufficient design of the facilities means social stress for cows which can be diminished by a high qualification of the herdsman to keep cattle. According to Tab. 1 we found a method to assess the herdsman's qualification.

TABLE 1    The Assessment of the Herdsman's Qualification
           to keep cattle. ( 15 points are the maximum ).
-----------------------------------------------------------

1. Handling
- calm handling
- ability to identify the individuals visually
- ability to assess the state of health of the individuals

2.State of the individual's maintenance
- care of the claws
- treatment of wounds
- care of the skin

3. Cleanness of the cow house
- feeding area
- walking area
- resting area

4. Handling of the livestock feeding
- feeding conform to the supply of feeding places
- species-specific quality of feed
- feeding at regular intervals

5 Handling of the cowshed equipment
- sufficient ventilation
- shoulder- and nose-rail conform to the animal's size
- immediate and competent repair of damaged facilities.

In 8 farms with a locomotion area of less than 3,6 m²/cow cattle with herdsmen of less than 12 qualification points showed a locomotion of more than 28 % than those with herdsmen of more than 12 points (Fig. 5). In 11 farms with a locomotion area of more than 3,6 m²/cow the difference of the cow's locomotion with herdsmen of different qualification was only 23 % (Fig. 6). In the cases with larger walking space a bad qualification of the herdsman had less influence to the locomotion of the cattle.

We found a high significant negativ correlation between

the qualification of the herdsmen and numbers of injuries in cattle : $r_s = -0,723$ (p <0,05), n = 10 farms.

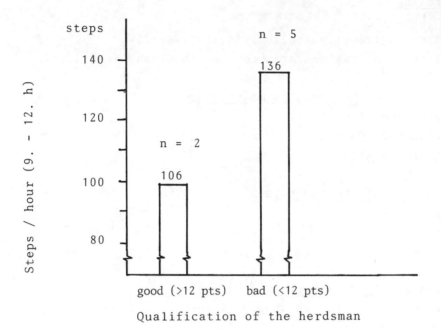

Fig. 5    Qualification of the herdsman and steps/hour on a walkingspace of <3,6 m²/cow.

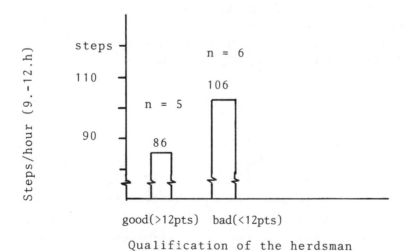

Fig. 6    Qualification of the herdsman and steps/hour on a walking space of >3,6 m²/cow.

CONCLUSION

Wiepkema (1985) stated : "When farm animals are brought into intensive husbandry systems ... density may be so high that for one or more behavioural states the interindividual distances become abnormally small. The animals involved will actively resist such a packed situation and if they have no success, stress will occur ..."

In our study we showed that insufficiency of walking space, number of feeding places and cubicles are stressing factors for cattle. They induce more social competition and more injuries in cattle. Furthermore bad qualification of the herdsman induces an increase of the effect of these factors.

According to this result social stress in cattle can be reduced in cubicle houses as follows:
- a minimum of a walking space of 3,5 $m^2$/cow
- at least one feeding place per cow
- at least one cubicle per cow
- improvement of the herdsman's qualification to keep cattle.

REFERENCE
WIEPKEMA, P.R.   1985. Control systems for coping at critical densities. In  "Social space for domestic animals". (Ed. R. Zayan). (Martinus Nijhoff, Dordrecht), p 237.

# EFFECTS OF AMPEROZIDE ON FIGHTING BEHAVIOUR AND ITS CONSEQUENCES ON PERFORMANCE IN PIGS

Anders K.K. Björk

Pharmacia LEO Therapeutics AB
P.O.Box 839, S-201 80  Malmö, Sweden

## ABSTRACT

Pigs fight vigorously as they establish a dominance
hierarchy. Fighting and a prolonged adaptation period cause
social stress that may adversely affect animal well-being.
A novel psychotropic drug, amperozide, when administered as
a single dose at mixing was found to substantially reduce
aggressive behaviour and, furthermore, to minimize long-term
negative effects on growth performance in both unacquainted
weanling and grower pigs. Pigs were penned in groups of 9 to
11 animals. The effect of amperozide on aggressive behaviour
and growth performance in restricted-fed 12-week-old pigs
was determined in a 4-week trial (Exp. 1). Injuries from
biting behaviour were reduced (P<0.001) in amperozide-
treated pigs compared with untreated controls (injury
scores: 1.16 vs 4.89 at 8 hours postpenning; 3.11 vs 7.98 at
48 hours). Social stability was reached within 48 hours.
Pigs were weighed on day 0, 3, 7 and 28. Amperozide-treated
pigs gained significantly more weight in each weighing
period up to 28 days. The improvement (P<0.001) in weight
gain on day 28 was 2.1 kg (18 %). When compared with
azaperone (Exp. 2), amperozide was found to be distinctly
superior in reducing aggressive behaviour. A series of
trials (Exp. 3) was conducted to determine the effect of
amperozide on weight gain of restricted-fed pigs during the
entire growing-finishing period. Untreated control pigs had
a poorer growth performance than did amperozide-treated
pigs. On an average, amperozide treatment improved (P<0.001)
average daily gain in the first 35 days postpenning by 91 g
(28 %). In 4-week-old pigs fed ad libitum (Exp. 4),
amperozide treatment had a substantial effect on average
daily gain during the entire 21-day trial period following
weaning. On an average, average daily gain was improved
(P<0.05) by 44 g (30 %) on day 21. Amperozide treatment did
not affect average daily feed intake. In the control group,
four pigs (10 %) died from diarrhoea during the first two
weeks of the trial. We conclude that there is a causal
association between social stress and long-term checks in
growth rate and gastrointestinal dysfunction following
weaning and mixing of pigs. By reducing excessive fighting,
amperozide decreases the adverse effects of social stress
upon regrouping.

INTRODUCTION

As a result of more intensive rearing and special-
ization in modern pig production, pigs are often mixed and
moved to a new location. Newly mixed pigs fight vigorously
as they establish a new dominance hierarchy. Fighting has
usually ceased and social stability may be observed within
24 to 48 hours of grouping (Ewbank, 1976; McGlone, 1986). It
is argued, however, that pig groups will not have adapted
completely to a new environment until several days after
introduction (Dantzer, 1973). This would suggest a catecholamine as well as a corticosteroid response to the stress
reaction following regrouping. The social stress following
mixing of unacquainted pigs may be the major contributor to
performance loss following regrouping (Björk et al., 1987).

Environmental parameters and management practices that
may affect the aggressive behaviour while hierarchy is being
established are not well known. Tranquillizers have been
used in attempts to control aggressive behaviour in pigs
but overall the beneficial effects of sedatives on pig
aggression are equivocal (Dantzer, 1974). However, one way
of reducing fighting when unacquainted pigs are placed together is to make the animals accustomed to each other in a
situation where serious conflict does not take place
(Fraser, 1984).

In the search for novel psychotropic agents, it is
recently demonstrated that amperozide (chemical name:
4-[4,4-bis(p-fluorophenyl)butyl]-N-ethyl-1-piperazine-
carboxamide) exhibited properties in rodents suggesting a
selective limbic profile of action. Thus, amperozide was
shown to affect emotional behaviours, i.e. to have anti-
aggressive and anticonflict properties. Contrary to
classical neuroleptics and anxiolytics, however, it did not
cause impairment of motor control or sedation. This promted
research to explore the use of amperozide as a possible way

to reduce fighting when unacquainted pigs are mixed together
and, furthermore, to determine long-term consequences of
aggressive behaviour on health and performance.


MATERIALS AND METHODS

Four experiments involving in total about 2000 pigs
were conducted. In Exp. 1 the effect of amperozide on agonistic behaviour and performance in restricted-fed grower
pigs was investigated. In Exp. 2 the effects of azaperone
(Stresnil, Janssen) and amperozide on agonistic behaviour in
weanling pigs were measured. Exp. 3 was designed to determine the effect of amperozide on weight gain in restricted-fed grower pigs and Exp. 4 to determine the effect of
amperozide on weight gain in weanling pigs when using ad
libitum feeding.

In all experiments Swedish Landrace x Yorkshire pigs
were used. The experiments were conducted in conventional
pig units. The grower pigs used were about 12 weeks of age
with an average body weight of about 22 kg. The weanling
pigs were about 5 weeks of age weighing about 8 kg. Pigs
were penned in groups of 9 to 11 animals, generally 10. Pens
provided 0.7 $m^2$ and 0.4 $m^2$ per pig of floor space for the
grower and weanling pigs, respectively. Treatments were
given either as a single intramuscular injection or as a
single oral administration immediately before or after
mixing. Restricted-fed pigs were all fed the same way
according to a pre-determined time-based scale with the
total daily allowance equally divided between two feedings.
A four-point scoring system was employed to evaluate degree
of physical damage from biting behaviour. The pig's body was
divided into six zones. A single observer noted the score of
injuries in each zone (based on the number of bite and slash
marks) for each individual pig immediately before penning
and  8, 26 and 48 hours postpenning. Analyses were performed
on the total of all scores.

For further details we are referring to the original papers (Björk et al., 1988; Björk, 1988).

RESULTS AND DISCUSSION

In Exp. 1, after a few minutes of exploratory behaviour following penning, fierce fighting involving biting and pushing episodes was recorded in the control pigs. The fighting was most intense the first four hours postpenning.

There were no fights recorded during the first six hours following penning in the amperozide-treated group. About 30 minutes after penning, the amperozide-treated pigs were seen to huddle together and lie on the top of one another. The pig groups stayed in this position for most of the first six hours. Pigs, however, were not sedated, because they remained responsive to handling procedures.

TABLE 1   Effects of amperozide on injury scores[a] recorded 0, 8, 26 and 48 hours after mixing (Exp. 1).

| Time, hours | Control | Amperozide |
|---|---|---|
| 0 | 0.01[b] | 0.07[b] |
| 8 | 4.89[b] | 1.16[c] |
| 26 | 7.43[b] | 2.27[c] |
| 48 | 7.98[b] | 3.11[c] |

[a]Injury scores on range 0 to 18
[b,c]Means in the same row with different superscripts differ (P<0.001)

Social stability, i.e. no fighting displayed, within the pig groups was reached at 48 hours. The number of bite and slash marks was significantly lower in the amperozide-treated pigs compared with the controls at 8, 26 and 48 hours after penning (Table 1).

Thus, amperozide was found not only to delay the initial violent aggressive outbursts but also to reduce the level of aggression subsequently. Hence, amperozide-treated pigs reached social stability with significantly less aggression and physical damage than the control pigs.

TABLE 2    Effects of azaperone and amperozide on injury scores[a] recorded 0, 8 and 26 hours after mixing (Exp. 2).

| Time, hours | Control | Azaperone | Amperozide |
|---|---|---|---|
| 0 | 0 | 0 | 0 |
| 8 | $4.5^{bx}$ | $3.0^{cx}$ | $0.2^{dy}$ |
| 26 | $5.2^{bex}$ | $3.6^{bexy}$ | $0.8^{cfy}$ |

[a] Injury scores on range 0 to 18
[b,c,d] Means in the same row with different superscripts differ ($P < 0.05$)
[e,f] Means in the same row with different superscripts differ ($P < 0.01$)
[x,y] Means in the same row with different superscripts differ ($P < 0.001$)

In Exp. 2, the effect of amperozide was compared with that of azaperone. In this trial, social stability was reached within 26 hours. The injury scores were significantly reduced at each time point in the amperozide-treated pigs compared with both controls and azaperone-treated pigs (Table 2). Azaperone-treated pigs had significantly fewer marks than the controls at 8 hours, but not at 26 hours postpenning. In effect, azaperone had a short-lasting sedative effect.

Results of studies on the effect of mixing pigs on weight gain have been contradictory. Previous workers, however, have usually found that regrouping reduces rate and efficiency of gain (Aherne, 1976; McGlone and Curtis, 1985; McGlone et al., 1986). Even though the cause-and-effect sequences have not been thoroughly analysed, marked alterations in the small intestinal structure and brush-border enzyme activities associated with a malabsorption syndrome have been reported in young pigs (Kenworthy, 1976; Hampson, 1986). A marked reduction of jejunal villous height at 3 and 7 days postweaning was found in both 21-day-old and 35-day-old weaned pigs. At 14 days postweaning, however, the villous height had lengthened (Cera et al., 1988).

TABLE 3    Effects of amperozide on weight gain during the first 4 weeks postpenning (Exp. 1).

| Initial weight, kg | Control | Amperozide |
|---|---|---|
| Initial weight, kg | 21.4 | 21.4 |
| Weight gain[a], kg | | |
| 0 - 3 days | -0.5[b] | 0.5[c] |
| 3 - 7 | 1.7[d] | 2.0[e] |
| 7 - 28 | 10.8[d] | 11.6[e] |

[a]Pigs were regrouped on day 1
[b,c]Means in the same row with different superscripts differ ($P < 0.001$)
[d,e]Means in the same row with different superscripts differ ($P < 0.05$)

In Exp. 1, the amperozide-treated pigs had gained significantly more weight than the control pigs when weighed on day 3, 7 and 28 postpenning (Table 3). The improvements in weight were 1.0 kg, 1.3 kg and 2.1 kg, respectively. Thus, amperozide-treated pigs had gained significantly more weight in each weighing period indicating a long-term check in growth rate after mixing.

TABLE 4   Effects of amperozide on average daily gain (g) in grower pigs during the first 5 weeks postpenning (Exp. 3).

| Trial No. | Control | Amperozide |
|-----------|---------|------------|
| 1 | 407 | 495 |
| 2 | 304 | 398 |
| 3 | 215 | 327 |
| 4 | 347 | 441 |
| 5 | 357 | 441 |
| 6 | 340 | 414 |

In Exp. 3, the effect of amperozide on weight gain was investigated in six different trials involving in total about 1600 pigs obtained at 20 to 25 kg live weight. Amperozide treatment improved ($P < 0.001$) average daily gain (ADG) in the first 35 days by 91 g (28 %) with an improvement of ADG of about the same order in all trials conducted (Table 4). This improvement (3.2 kg) was found to persist through to slaughter (2.6 kg).

TABLE 5    Effects of amperozide on performance in
           weanling pigs during the first 3 weeks
           postpenning (Exp. 4).

| Parameter | Control | Amperozide |
|---|---|---|
| Avg daily gain, g | | |
| 0 - 4 days | $15^a$ | $58^b$ |
| 4 - 7 | $50^a$ | $97^b$ |
| 7 - 14 | $129^a$ | $173^b$ |
| 14 - 21 | $276^a$ | $317^a$ |
| 0 - 21 | $144^a$ | $188^b$ |
| Avg daily feed, kg | | |
| 0 - 4 days | 0.22 | 0.20 |
| 4 - 7 | 0.25 | 0.25 |
| 7 - 14 | 0.40 | 0.40 |
| 14 - 21 | 0.62 | 0.56 |

[a,b] Means in the same row with different superscripts
      differ (P<0.05)

In weanling pigs (Exp. 4), the amperozide treatment had
a substantial effect on ADG during the entire 21-day trial
period postweaning. Amperozide-treated pigs gained (P<0.05)
more weight during each weighing period in the 0- to 14-day
period and had gained (P<0.05) 0.9 kg (30 %) more weight
when weighed on day 21. Average daily feed intake was not
affected by the amperozide treatment. In the control group,
pigs were temporarily affected by severe postweaning
diarrhoea. Though adequate antimicrobial treatment was given

four pigs (10 %) died during the first 14 days of the trial.
No pig was severely affected by diarrhoea in the amperozide
treated group.

Whatever the ultimate cause to the poor performance in
control pigs following regrouping, the precipitating factor
is believed to have been the mixing of pigs. The results of
the trials presented would suggest that the excessive fighting during establishment of a dominance hierarchy led to a
detrimental adaptation process, causing a longer and more
adverse effect on feed efficiency, and hence ɟrowth performance, than would be expected generally.

In the physical sense, the pen is a restricted community in that its members are confined together and are
thus forced to associate. It is reasonable to presume that
the level of aggression is even higher in a restricted
rather than an unrestricted environment because confinement puts a restraint on flight-related behaviours.

If the stress of a single traumatic experiences is of
sufficient magnitude, one-trial conditioning will occur and
the original anxiety and its autonomic concomitant may be
trigged again by any reminder or even a threat of the
circumstances which occurred at the time of the original
trauma (Kelly, 1980). With repeated exposure to the reminder, however, the adverse effect will usually subside
over a period of time. We now argue that one-trial conditioning in pigs may occur as a consequence to the fierce
fighting displayed when unfamiliar pigs in larger groups are
brought together, with the reminder being a dominant
pen-mate (Ewbank and Meese, 1971).

An animal that perceives itself being unable to control
its surroundings shows a dramatic increase in adrenocortical
activity while exposed to such conditions (Levine, 1985).
Indeed, the level of circulating corticosteroids was reported to be higher when pigs engaged in aggressive behaviour.

Moreover, the mere presence of a dominant pig, when perceived as a threat, led to increased pituitary-adrenal
activity (Arnone and Dantzer, 1980). Furthermore, it has
been found that stimuli which are perceived as stressful can
modulate the immune response (Ader, 1981; Lloyd, 1987). A
reduced villous height was found in wasting (unthrifty) pigs
probably suffering from chronic social stress (Jönsson and
Martinsson, 1976; Martinsson et al., 1976). An increased
susceptibility to infectious diseases, such as coliform
enteritis, is one of the most characteristic features of the
postweaning period (Fraser et al., 1975). This implies a
causal association between social stress from agonistic
behaviour and maladaptation, and poor growth and disease. A
single amperozide treatment at mixing would have a favourable effect on the adaptation process thereby reducing the
social stress reaction on the concomitant behavioural and
neuroendocrine responses.

ACKNOWLEDGEMENTS

I am greatly indebted to Nils-Göran Olsson for his
skilled technical assistance. I wish to thank Professor
Kjell Martinsson for his advice and guidance, and
Maj-Lis Brandt for typing the manuscript.

REFERENCES

Ader, R. (Editor). 1981. Psychoneuroimmunology. Academic
    Press, New York, pp. 661.
Aherne, F.X. 1976. Feeding and management of the weaned pig.
    55th Annu. Feeders Day Rep. Univ. of Alberta, Edmonton,
    pp. 63-65.
Arnone, M. and Dantzer, R. 1980. Does frustration induce
    aggression in pigs? Appl. Anim. Ethol., 6, 351-362.
Björk, A.K.K. 1988. Is social stress in pigs a detrimental
    factor to health and growth that can be avoided by
    amperozide treatment? Appl. Anim. Behav. Sci., sub-
    mitted.
Björk, A.K.K., Olsson, N.-G.E., Martinsson, K.B. and
    Göransson, L.A.T. 1987. A note on the role of be-
    haviour in pig production and the effect of
    amperozide on growth performance. Anim. Prod., 45,
    523-526.

Björk, A., Olsson, N.-G., Christensson, E., Martinsson, K. and Olsson, O. 1988. Effects of amperozide on biting behavior and performance in restricted-fed pigs following regrouping. J. Anim. Sci., 66, 669-675.

Cera, K.R., Mahan, D.C., Cross, R.F., Reinhardt, G.A. and Whitmoyer, R.E. 1988. Effect of age, weaning and post-weaning diet on the small intestinal growth and jenunal morphology in young swine. J. Anim. Sci., 66, 574-584.

Dantzer, R. 1973. Étude de la stabilisation des rythmes d'activité locomotrice de porcelets introduits dans un nouvel environnment. J. Physiol. Paris, 66, 495-503.

Dantzer, R. 1974. Les tranquillisants en elevage: Revue critique. Ann. Rech. Vet., 5, 465-505.

Ewbank, R. 1976. Social hierarchy in suckling and fattening pigs: A review. Livest. Prod. Sci., 3, 363-372.

Ewbank, R. and Meese, G.B. 1971. Aggressive behaviour in groups of domesticated pigs on removal and return of individuals. Anim. Prod., 13, 685-693.

Fraser, D. 1984. The role of behavior in swine production: a review of research. Appl. Anim. Ethol. 11, 317-339.

Fraser, D., Ritchie, J.S.D. and Fraser, A.F. 1975. The term "stress" in the veterinary context. Brit. Vet. J., 131, 653-663.

Hampson, D.J. 1986. Alterations in piglet small intestinal structure at weaning. Res. Vet. Sci., 40, 32-40.

Jönsson, L. and Martinsson, K. 1976. Regional ileitis in pigs. Morphological and pathogenetical aspects. Acta Vet. Scand., 17, 223-232.

Kelly, D. (Editor), 1980. The effect of conditioning in man and animals. In Anxiety and Emotions. Charles C. Thomas Publisher, Springfield, Illinois, pp. 49-60.

Kenworthy, R. 1976. Observations on the effects of weaning in the young pig. Clinical and histopathological studies of intestinal function and morphology. Res. Vet. Sci., 21, 69-75.

Levine, S. 1975. A definition of stress? In: G.P. Moberg (Editor), Animal Stress. Amer. Physiol. Soc., Bethesda, Maryland, pp. 51-70.

Lloyd, R. (Editor) 1987. Explorations in psychoneuroimmunology. Grune & Stratton, Inc., Orlando, Florida, pp. 126.

Martinsson, K., Ekman, K. and Jönsson, L. 1976. Hematological and biochemical analyses of blood and serum in pigs with regional ileitis with special reference to the pathogenesis. Acta Vet. Scand., 17, 233-243.

McGlone, J.J. 1986. Influence of resources on pig aggression and dominance. Behav. Processes, 12, 135-144.

McGlone, J.J. and Curtis, S.E. 1985. Behavior and performance of weanling pigs in pens equipped with hide areas. J. Anim. Sci., 60, 20-24.

McGlone, J.J., Stansbury, W.F. and Tribble, L.F. 1986. Aerosolized 5α-androst-16-en-3-one reduced agonist behavior and temporarily improved performance of growing pigs. J. Anim. Sci., 63, 679-684.

FINAL DISCUSSION AND CONCLUSIONS

COMMISSION OF THE EUROPEAN COMMUNITIES

COMMUNITY PROGRAMME FOR THE CO-ORDINATION OF AGRICULTURAL RESEARCH


SOCIAL STRESS IN FARM ANIMALS

MAY 26-27, 1988

BRUSSELS, BELGIUM.


FINAL DISCUSSION

REPORT BY MARTIN MURPHY

(AIDED BY YVES LAMBERTY, JEFF RUSHEN AND ANDREW MILLS).


## INTRODUCTION

The report which follows outlines the basic concepts and
principles which were discussed at a meeting on social stress in
farm animals. While the major part of the text deals with the
final discussion session, where appropriate, relevant sections
from other discussion sessions are included.

## SOCIAL STRESS ( DEFINITIONS AND ASSESSMENT )

During the course of the meeting social stress was defined in
terms of adrenocorticoid measures (figure 1), aggressive
interactions, isolation and the response state of the animal
resulting from social stressors. The classical hormones to
evaluate when considering stress have been the glucocorticoids
(cortisol, in particular) and the catecholamines (epinephrine and
norepinephrine). There is however, a critical need to evalute
hormonal measurements with behavioural, immunological and
ecological correlates so that a complete picture of a "stressful"

295

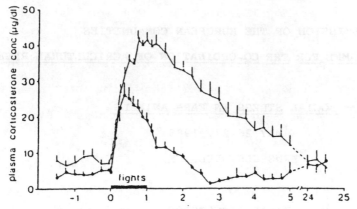

Figure 1. Plasma corticosterone concentrations of victors (n = 6, ●) and losers (n = 9, ▲) during and after the 1-hours fight. Bars = SEM (after Schuurman, 1984).

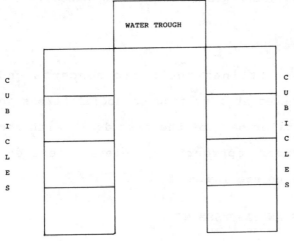

Figure 2. Location of a water trough in a blind alley in a cubicle house for dairy cows which will lead to aggresive interactions due to crowding.

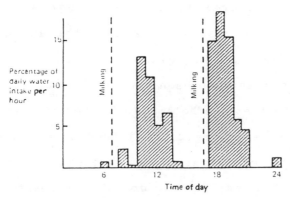

Figure 3. Herd drinking pattern in winter (MAFF, 1986).

situation can be interpreted accurately. The word "stress" is a upsetting to many people. If an animal is in a state of uncertainty or if predictability or controllability over the environment changes then we may regard the animal as "stressed". However, the ability of an animal to respond to stressors indicates that it has some controllability over its environment. If social stress is measured in terms of the classic neuroendocrinological responses, how differently does the animal react when it is confronted by other inert stressors such as heat, cold or electric shock. "Stress" per se is a non-specific process hence the responses seen are always going to be similar.

**FAMILIARITY PROCESSES**

Social stability will exist in a group of animals if the animals can predict changes in the environment and if animals have a lot of information about each other that is familiarity exists in the social group. When talking about social stress, it is important to talk in terms of relationships between individuals and in this context "the pair" is the simplest model to use. How do animals gain information about conspecifics ? To answer this question we need to know more about familiarity processes in animals. It is easy to classify crowding and aggresion as social stressors. A more detailed analysis of animal production in general will show that in current systems of rearing livestock, animals such as dairy cows are kept in unnatural social groups, and the weaning of calves of dairy cows is carried out at very unnatural times. From these two examples it is obvious that our concept of social stress should not be limited to aggressive interactions but that a broader view of the concept should be taken.

## SOCIAL IGNORANCE

It is possible that one of the consequences of current rearing systems will be to prevent the development of social characteristics. At this point the term "social ignorance" should be introduced. This refers to the situation which is well described in pigs (Schouten, 1986) where failure of the young pigs to undergo a losing experience, or to learn about losing, could have disastrous consequences for its health and well-being if it engages in conflict with an older pig for the first time. Ideally, one could then say that animals should be reared in situations for which they have evolved. While this concept is important, one should remember that some current methods of housing animals do not fulfill the "ethological needs" of animals as we determine them.

Social stress implies a lack of functioning of the social system. Co-operation between individuals is fundamental for the formation of a social system. But for animals to co-operate there must be by definition familiarity between conspecifics. Another component of the social stress picture is that in the wild, social instability rarely occurs. There are two possible explanations for these phenomena: a) in unconfined situations there is a large area available to the animals, hence the likelihood of them meeting a conspecific is reduced and b) if an aggressive interaction does occur then the loser has a larger area to escape into. Although animals have evolved into a social structure in which aggressive behaviour is not common, the problems of aggresive interactions (or fighting) which are seen in current systems of production are management-induced.

In macaques and baboons, aggressive interactions between conspecifics are rare. This is due to fact that the group structure of these animals is based on lateral social pressure. In this situation, it is possible to predict what the dominant animal is going to do and therefore one can avoid or minimise confrontation. The ability to focalise attention on the likely activities of the dominant animal in the group helps to maintain stability. In contrast to primates where facial expressions, postures, smells and so on are easy to understand, the idea of being able to interpret such messages from pigs, sheep or cattle is not possible as yet. Hence, phylogenetically low or high animals are therefore easier to study and understand when we are trying to evaluate social stress.

Just as it is important to observe the animals in any social stress study, it is essential that we do not overlook the ecological situation within which these animals are placed or are naturally living in. A good example of this interaction is seen in Antechinus, a marsupial (Bradley, McDonald and Lee, 1980) where males only live for three weeks after they reach maturity. They then attempt to kill each other. Those animals that die show all the characteristics of a typical chronic stress situation that is, stomach wall ulceration , heart damage and enlarged adrenal glands. In any social group the better that animals know each other, the better will be the communication, in a ritualised manner, between the members of that group. This highlights once again the importance of familiarity in a social system as a means of reducing and preventing aggressive interactions. Further research into the "natural" structure of a species will help to give us clearer insights into the ways in which animals regulate their behaviour when in particular social systems. The study of the ontogeny of various behaviours in "natural" ecological situations will also help to contribute to a more complete understanding of animal behaviour in non-confinement situations.

## GENETICS AND SOCIAL STRESS

What role does genetics have to play in the responses of animals to stressors ? First of all, it is obvious that a wide range of genotypes is present in any species. Secondly, based on the fact that a diversity of genotypes is obvious, we must then address the question of what causes a stereotypic behaviour or adrenocortical response to differ between animals. In other words, what is causing individual variation between animals? If there are environments where animals have adapted successfully, then these situations need close examination to elucidate a) why the animal succeeded in adapting and b) what components of that environment facilitate adaptation over others. Genetic selection of animals can take place in a given direction once we know the characteristics that we wish to select for. It may be possible to select for breeds which show reduced aggression but in so doing we may affect growth rate, for example. The genetic factors controlling aggression in animals , the genetic coding or DNA sequences involved must be elucidated as one component of the mechanisms of aggression in animals.

## STOCKMANSHIP AND MINIMISING SOCIAL STRESS

In this context, it may be worth looking at the role that the stockman has to play in keeping his charges content or reducing social stress. Habituation of the animals to their caretaker may help to reduce fear in the animals and this will be seen as reduced flight distance. In dairy cows , for example, if the farmer talks to his cows, if he handles them gently in the milking parlour and most importantly if he handles/manages them well as calves this should result in quiet heifers when the animals subsequently calve down. It has been shown in rats for example that gentle handling of the young pups will render them more friendly towards humans. This is manifest as reduced heart rate in the pups accustomed to handling (Denenberg, 1964, 1967). In other words they react less to stressful situations both behaviourally and hormonally. Behaviourally this is manifest as better avoidance (Doty and O'Hare, 1966) with a concommitant lower corticosterone response (Ader, 1968). The consequences of rough handling of dairy cows may be increased flight distance and perhaps unstable group hierarchies. Stressful stimuli in dairy cows can induce the release of epinephrine and norepinephrine which cause vasoconstriction (that is reduced blood supply) and reduce the amount of oxytocin reaching the myoepithelial cells in the mammary gland (Chan, 1965). This may result in reduced milk yield. In any situation where man is dealing with animals it is essential that constancy of approach/handling exists. It could be argued that stockmen are not always consistent in their management of animals and that perhaps robotic systems of for example milking cows will provide that consistency of approach. Other advantages of computerisation of dairy cow management systems is that oestrus detection efficiency, mastitis control and general cow health could be assessed more accurately. This can ultimately lead to an improvement in the cow's welfare, minimise the potentially stressful effect of the stockman and increase production efficiency.

## POTENTIAL WAYS OF REDUCING SOCIAL STRESS IN ANIMALS

A number of options are available to reduce or minimise social stress in animals. We can a) manipulate the animal's nervous system or b) alter the animal's environment and therefore its' behaviour.

## PHARMACOLOGICAL CONTROL OF SOCIAL STRESS IN FARM ANIMALS

Taking the problem of social stress to a practical level, what does a farmer do to minimise the economic consequences of fighting amongst a group of pigs. Firstly, mixing of pigs should be avoided, but this is not always possible. Secondly, trying to keep pigs of similar weights together should help to minimise the attack of lower animals in the social group. However, this is not always a practical proposition. A third approach which can be considered is to use neuroleptics which are drugs producing a state in which the animal, although semi-conscious, remains in whatever position it is placed (Brander, Pugh and Bywater, 1982). Neuroleptics such as azaperone or amperozide act to reduce sensory perception and thereby tranquilise the animal. Treatment of animals at potentially "stressful" times such as mixing will help to prevent and reduce aggressive behaviour. Therapeutic regimes exist therefore to reduce social stress. It could be argued that we are merely treating the external signs of social stress when we advocate the use of tranquilisers and that the causal factor(s) still escape us. This is true. However, it should not prevent future research from looking at the mechanisms of social stress, cues used by animals and so on. But what do farmers do when they are waiting for this information on methods of reducing social stress to be developed ? Pharmacological manipulation of the central nervous system using tranquilisers is a practical means of controlling social stress. The problem of residues in meat and consumer awareness of same might influence the future use of these compounds.

The social organisation of animals is adaptible. It is possible that the animals in current production systems are now at the limit of their adaptabilities. Our aim should now be to try to help animals adapt at different levels to their envirionment. This may involve providing substrate such as straw to animals to keep them occupied. Animals adapt through learning or ontogenetically. Based on this, future research should be directed at how animals adapt and consequently how we can help them when they are placed in environments not conducive to their welfare.

## MANIPULATION OF THE ANIMALS' ENVIRONMENT

Some of the conventional methods of housing farm animals have detrimental effects on the well-being of the animal occupants. This reduced welfare can manifest as lameness in dairy cows to cannibalistic behaviour in battery cage hens. Housing type and layout can influence the occurence of social stress in animals. If stocking density for example is too high, the inter-individual distances between animals will be reduced. The likelihood of confrontation increases and group stability consequently will be reduced. Improper housing design can lead to excessive aggressive interactions. A simple example is shown in figure 2. In this example the water trough is found in a blind alley. At peak times during the day, such as after milking and in the afternoon between 3pm and 9pm (figure 3) cows have their highest water requirement (MAFF, 1986). If the water source is located in a blind alley, crowding will occur and fighting may result. Strategic placing of the water supply in an area where congestion is less likely to occur will reduce the incidence of aggressive interactions.

It is prudent at this point to introduce a note of caution. At present much research is being carried out on alternative housing systems for livestock (mainly laying hens, veal calves and tethered sows). Most of this research revolves around designing less intensive housing systems wherein species such as laying hens are placed. When, or if the system does not work, the housing layout is altered as a means of making the system work efficiently. This approach is a little foolhardy. The more logical approach to designing alternative housing for animals is first to examine the behaviour of the animals, to quantify the "needs" viz for bedding, feed preference and so on and then to design accomodation which allows the animals to engage in those behaviour patterns which research has identified as being "needs" or essential for the welfare of the animals. The provision of hideaways offers some means of escape from attack for lower members of a social group. In a similar manner toys or substrates which enrich the environment help to alter the animals' perception of the environment and in so doing may reduce social stress.

**CONCLUSIONS**

To date, there have been no experiments which have been precise enough to define the social or individual components of a stressor. Future experiments in the area of social stress must be carefully designed and variables in the environment must be defined and assessed accordingly.

Continued research into the mechanisms of familiarity processes, social recognition, coping strategies and so on must not be abandoned if information is to be generated about the organisation of social groups of animals. This information will help designers of animal accomodation and legislators to provide guidelines on the housing of animals which will minimise the potentially negative effects of social stress.

More information is required on how to best assess or quantify stress in animals. It is clear that an integrated approach using neuroendocrine, ethological, immunological and ecological information offers the best approach.

A lot of emphasis in applied ethological studies is placed on the negative aspects of social behaviour such as aggression and fighting and to neglect the more positive aspects such as association and synchronisation. Social animals tend to synchronise their activities and to stay in close proximity (Dantzer, 1985). Investigations into the mechanisms of social cohesion should form a major part of social stress research in the future.

## REFERENCES

Ader, R. (1968). Effects of early experience on emotional and physiological reactivity. J.Comp. Physiol. Psychol. 66:264-271.

Bradley, A.J., McDonald, I.R.M. and Lee, A.K. (1980). Stress and mortality in a small marsupial (Antechinus stuartii, Mcleay). Gen. Comp. Endocrinol. 40: 188-

Brander, G.C., Pugh, M.P. and Bywater, R.J. (1982). Veterinary Applied Pharmacology and Therapeutics. Chapter 4th edition. Balliere Tindall, London.

Chan, Y. (1965). Mechanism of epinephrine inhibition of the milk-ejecting response to oxytocin. J. Pharmacol. Exp. Ther. 147: 48 - 56.

Dantzer, R. (1985). Applied ethological research on farm animals other than poultry: An introduction. In: Social Space for Domestic Animals. Edited by R. Zayan. Current Topics in Veterinary Medicine and Animal Science, Number 35. Martinus Nijhoff, pp 114 - 115.

Denenberg, V.H. (1964). Critical periods, stimulus input and emotional reactivity: A theory of infantile stimulation. Psychology Reviews. 71, 335 - 342.

Denenberg, V.H. (1967). Stimulation in infancy, emotional reactivity, and exploratory behaviour. In: Neurophysiology and Emotion. Edited by D.C. Glass. The Rockerfeller University Press and Russel Sage Foundation, p61.

Doty, B.A. and O'Hare, K.M. (1966). Interaction of shock intensity, age, and handling offoots of avoidance conditioning. Perceptual and Motor Skills 23: 1311-1322.

MAFF, (1986). Drinking water for dairy cows. Leaflet 634. Ministry of Agriculture, Fisheries and Food, Lion House, Willowburn Estate, Alnwick, Northumberland, NE66 2PF.

Schouten, W.G.P. (1986). Rearing conditions and Behaviour in Pigs. PhD thesis, Agricultural University, Wageningen.

Schuurman, T. (1984). Endocrine processes underlying victory and defeat in the male rat. Thesis State University Groningen, The Netherlands.

# LIST OF PARTICIPANTS

BELGIUM

Dr M. HERREMANS

Fysiologie der Huisdieren
Katholieke Universiteit Leuven
K. Mercierlaan 92
B-3030 Heverlee

Dr Y. LAMBERTY

Unité de Psychobiologie
Université Catholique de Louvain
Place Croix du Sud 1
B-1348 Louvain-la-Neuve

Dr F. ODBERG

Laboratorium voor Veetelt
Rijksuniversiteit Gent
Heidestraat 19
B-9220 Merelbeke

Dr R. ZAYAN

Unité de Psychobiologie
Université Catholique de Louvain
Place Croix du Sud 1
B-1348 Louvain-la-Neuve


DENMARK

Dr L.J. LYDEHOJ

Department of Research in
Pigs and Horses
National Institute of Animal Science
Postboks 39
DK-8833 Orum Sonderlyng

Dr M. HAGELSO

Department of Research in
Pigs and Horses
National Institute of Animal Science
Postboks 39
DK-8833 Orum Sonderlyng

Dr L. MUNKSGAARD

Department of Research in
Cattle and Sheep
National Institute of Animal Science
Postboks 39
DK-8833 Orum Sonderlyng

FEDERAL REPUBLIC OF GERMANY

Dr J. LADEWIG

Institut fur Tierzucht und
Tierverhalten - FAL
Institutsteil Trenthorst/Wulmenau
D-2061 Westerau 2

Dr J. RUSHEN

Wohnheim Goethe-Institut
Zimmer 211
Agnesstrasse 11
D-8000 Munchen 40

Dr K. ZEEB

Tierhygienisches Institut Freiburg
Am Moosweiher 2
D-7800 Freiburg

GREECE

Dr C. SPYRAKI

Department of Pharmacology
National University of Athens
Medical School
Goudi
11527 Athens

FRANCE

Dr M.F. BOUISSOU

INRA
Station de Physiologie Animale
Nouzilly (Tours)
37380 Monnaie

Dr R. DANTZER

INSERM Unité 259
Domaine de Carreire
Rue Camille Saint-Saëns
33077 Bordeaux

Dr J.M. FAURE

INRA
Station de Recherches Avicoles
Nouzilly (Tours)
37380 Monnaie

Dr A. MILLS

INRA
Station de Recherches Avicoles
Nouzilly (Tours)
37380 Monnaie

Dr P. MORMEDE

INSERM Unité 259
Domaine de Carreire
Rue Camille Saint-Saëns
33077 Bordeaux

Dr M.C. SALAUN

INRA
Station de Recherches sur
l'Elevage des Porcs
35590 L'Hermitage (Rennes)

Dr I. VEISSIER

INRA
Station des Productions
Bovines et Chevalines
Theix
63122 Ceyrat


IRELAND

Dr M. MURPHY

Department of Animal Husbandry
Faculty of Veterinary Medicine
University College
Ballsbridge
Dublin 4


ITALY

Dr A. BALDI

Istituto di Zootecnica Veterinaria
Universita di Milano
Via Celoria 10
20133 Milano

Dr E. CANALI

Istituto per la Difensa e
Valorizzazione del
Germoplasma Animale
Facolta di Medicina Veterinaria
CNR
Via Celoria 10
Milano


NETHERLANDS

Dr W.G.P. SCHOUTEN

Agricultural University
Department of Animal Husbandry
and Ethology
Marijkeweg 40
6709 PG Wageningen

Dr P.R. WIEPKEMA                    Agricultural University
                                    Department of Animal Husbandry
                                    and Ethology
                                    Marijkeweg 40
                                    6709 PG Wageningen

Dr H.K. WIERENGA                    Research Institute for
                                    Animal Production
                                    Schoonord. PO Box 501
                                    3700 AM Zeist


PORTUGAL


Dr J. SALAVESSA                     Escola Superior de Medicina
                                    Veterinaria
                                    Rua Gomes Freire
                                    1100 Lisboa


SPAIN


Dr V. GAUDIOSO                      Departamento de Produccion Animal
                                    Universidad de Leon
                                    Campus de la Vegazana
                                    24007 Leon


UNITED KINGDOM


Dr P.F. BRAIN                       Biological Sciences
                                    University College of Swansea
                                    Swansea, SA2 8PP
                                    Wales

Dr I.J.H. DUNCAN                    AFRC. Institute of Animal
                                    Physiology and Genetics Research
                                    Edinburgh Research Station
                                    Roslin
                                    Midlothian EH25 9PS
                                    Scotland

Dr K. KENDRICK                      AFRC. Institute of Animal
                                    Physiology and Genetics Research
                                    Cambridge Research Station
                                    Babraham Hall
                                    Cambridge CB2 4AT
                                    England

Dr R.F. PARROTT

AFRC. Institute of Animal
Physiology and Genetics Research
Cambridge Research Station
Babraham Hall
Cambridge CB2 4AT
England

Dr M. SEABROOK

Department of Agriculture and
Horticulture
University of Nottingham
Sutton Bonington
Loughborough
Leics LE12 5RD
England

Dr C. TERLOW

The East of Scotland College
of Agriculture
Animal Production Advisory and
Development Department
Bush Estate, Penicuik
Midlothian EH26 0QE
Scotland

ADDITIONAL PARTICIPANTS

Dr A. BJORK

AB Ferrosan
PO Box 839
S-20180 Malmo
SWEDEN

Dr J.J. Mc GLONE

Department of Animal Science
Texas Tech University
Lubbock, TX 79409-2141
U.S.A.

Dr J. CONNELL

Commission of the European
Communities DG VI
Rue de la Loi 200
B-1049 Brussels
BELGIUM

# Current Topics in Veterinary Medicine and Animal Science

Recent publications

**1984**

26. Manipulation of Growth in Farm Animals, edited by J.F. Roche and D. O'Callaghan. ISBN 0–89838–617–8
27. Latent Herpes Virus Infections in Veterinary Medicine, edited by G. Wittmann, R.M. Gaskell and H.-J. Rziha. ISBN 0–89838–622–5
28. Grassland Beef Production, edited by W. Holmes. ISBN 0–89838–650–0
29. Recent Advances in Virus Diagnosis, edited by M.S. McNulty and J.B. McFerran. ISBN 0–89838–674–8
30. The Male in Farm Animal Reproduction, edited by M. Courot. ISBN 0–89838–682–9

**1985**

31. Endocrine Causes of Seasonal and Lactational Anestrus in Farm Animals, edited by F. Ellendorff and F. Elsaesser. ISBN 0–89838–738–8
32. Brucella Melitensis, edited by J.M. Verger and M. Plommet. ISBN 0–89838–742–6

**1986**

33. Diagnosis of Mycotoxicoses, edited by J.L. Richard and J.R. Thurston. ISBN 0–89838–751–5
34. Embryonic Mortality in Farm Animals, edited by J.M. Sreenan and M.G. Diskin. ISBN 0–89838–772–8
35. Social Space for Domestic Animals, edited by R. Zayan. ISBN 0–89838–773–6
36. The Present State of Leptospirosis Diagnosis and Control, edited by W.A. Ellis and T.W.A. Little. ISBN 0–89838–777–9
37. Acute Virus Infections of Poultry, edited by J.B. McFerran and M.S. McNulty. ISBN 0–89838–809–0

**1987**

38. Evaluation and Control of Meat Quality in Pigs, edited by P.V. Tarrant, G. Eikelenboom and G. Monin. ISBN 0–89838–854–6
39. Follicular Growth and Ovulation Rate in Farm Animals, edited by J.F. Roche and D. O'Callaghan. ISBN 0–89838–855–4
40. Cattle Housing Systems, Lameness and Behaviour, edited by H.K. Wierenga and D.J. Peterse. ISBN 0–89838–862–7
41. Physiological and Pharmacological Aspects of the Reticulo-rumen, edited by L.A.A. Ooms, A.D. Degryse and A.S.J.P.A.M. van Miert. ISBN 0–89838–878–3
42. Biology of Stress in Farm Animals: An Integrative Approach, edited by P.R. Wiepkema and P.W.M. van Adrichem. ISBN 0–89838–895–3
43. Helminth Zoonoses, edited by S. Geerts, V. Kumar and J. Brandt. ISBN 0–89838–896–1
44. Energy Metabolism in Farm Animals: Effects of Housing, Stress and Disease, edited by M.W.A. Verstegen and A.M. Henken. ISBN 0–89838–974–7
45. Summer Mastitis, edited by G. Thomas, H.J. Over, U. Vecht and P. Nansen. ISBN 0–89838–982–8

**1988**

46. Modelling of Livestock Production Systems, edited by S. Korver and J.A.M. van Arendonk. ISBN 0–89838–373–0
47. Increasing Small Ruminant Productivity in Semi-arid Areas, edited by E.F. Thomson and F.S. Thomson. ISBN 0–89838–386–2
48. The Management and Health of Farmed Deer, edited by H.W. Reid. ISBN 0–89838–408–7

**1989**

49. Vaccination and Control of Aujeszky's Disease, edited by J.T. van Oirschot. ISBN 0–7923–0184–6
50. Pathological Histology of Domestic Animals, edited by J. von Sandersleben, K. Dämmrich and E. Dahme. ISBN 0–7923–0311–3
51. Diagnostic Ultrasound and Animal Reproduction, edited by M.A.M. Taverne and A.H. Willemse. ISBN 0–7923–0403–9
52. Improving Genetic Disease Resistance on Farm Animals, edited by A.J. van der Zijpp and W. Sybesma. ISBN 0–7923–0518–3